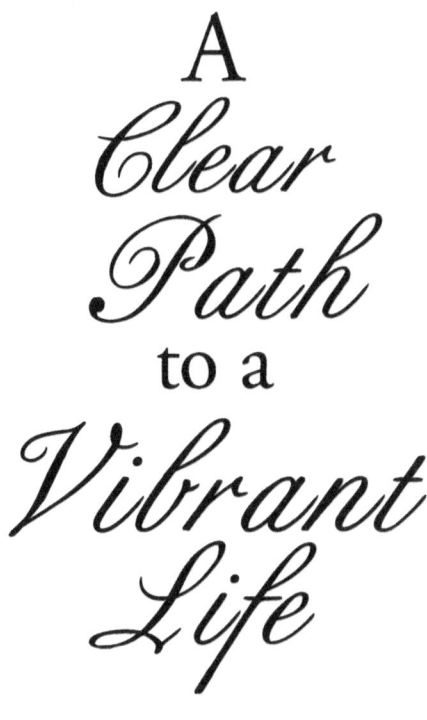

A Clear Path to a Vibrant Life

7 SIMPLE STEPS TO INCREASE YOUR
ENERGY AND HAPPINESS!

DONNA PARKER, L.Ac.

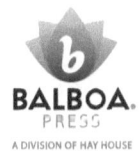

BALBOA.
PRESS
A DIVISION OF HAY HOUSE

Balboa Press books may be ordered through booksellers or by contacting:

Balboa Press
A Division of Hay House
1663 Liberty Drive
Bloomington, IN 47403
www.balboapress.com
1 (877) 407-4847

Because of the dynamic nature of the Internet, any web addresses or links contained in this book may have changed since publication and may no longer be valid. The views expressed in this work are solely those of the author and do not necessarily reflect the views of the publisher, and the publisher hereby disclaims any responsibility for them.

The author of this book does not dispense medical advice or prescribe the use of any technique as a form of treatment for physical, emotional, or medical problems without the advice of a physician, either directly or indirectly. The intent of the author is only to offer information of a general nature to help you in your quest for emotional and spiritual well-being. In the event you use any of the information in this book for yourself, which is your constitutional right, the author and the publisher assume no responsibility for your actions.

Any people depicted in stock imagery provided by Thinkstock are models, and such images are being used for illustrative purposes only.
Certain stock imagery © Thinkstock.

Print information available on the last page.

ISBN: 978-1-5043-6109-5 (sc)
ISBN: 978-1-5043-6110-1 (hc)
ISBN: 978-1-5043-6111-8 (e)

Library of Congress Control Number: 2016910484

Balboa Press rev. date: 10/31/2016

TABLE OF CONTENTS
Seven Steps in Seven Weeks

INTRODUCTION

Who Am I, and What Is My Story?

I'm "that" mom at school who doesn't like cupcakes served in the classroom at 10 a.m. My interest in health and fitness dates back to the 1970s when I did yoga as a kid back when only hippies did it. As a teenager, I read *Prevention* magazine and spent Saturday mornings watching PBS cooking shows. But I was also the kid who loved sugar and all things sweet. As a way to feed my sugar addiction, I became a very good baker at a young age. It was the best way to keep a steady flow of carbs and sugar in my life. Things have changed around my house, but I still love to bake. I just don't do it weekly, and when I do, I use ingredients that are healthier than white flour and refined sugar.

I coach people about healthy eating and healthy living. I help them with their health issues and work with them to figure out ways they can transform damaging habits into healthy ones without feeling deprived. That's the purpose of this workbook. I wanted something that would be easy for people to do. I hope you find this information not only helpful but also useful in your everyday life.

How to Use This Workbook

Each week I'll cover a new topic. Read through the week's topic and then, one at a time, start adding the concepts discussed to your life during that week. For example, Week 1 covers intention, meditation, and self-limiting beliefs. Start by setting your intentions, and then, a day or so later, add meditation. Finally, set aside some time to explore your self-limiting beliefs.

At the end of each week, you'll see a list of weekly reflections. Take a few minutes to rate how you're feeling. This exercise will help you keep track of the changes you are making as the weeks go by.

WEEK 1

Setting Yourself Up For Success

How to Change

Have you ever noticed how hard change can be? Doing things like getting off sugar or coffee or exercising more can just add stress to your life. And when it's not easy, you don't stick with it.

What many people don't realize is that a one-degree change can put you in an entirely different place in a very short time. Think about a ship heading from New York to Spain. Where might that ship end up if it was one degree off course? Perhaps Morocco! That's a big difference. Now picture yourself making a one-degree change in your life. Where might you end up six months or a year from now?

Stanford researcher B. J. Fogg discovered that behavior is systematic. That is, we don't change our behavior through sheer willpower. To make lasting changes in your behavior, you need three components: motivation, ability, and a trigger event.

What does that mean? Consider the following situation. You want to lose weight. That's your intention. What's your motivation? You want to be able to keep up with your kids. Not eating daily dessert is the ability. Not buying dessert when grocery shopping is the trigger event, allowing you to keep your intention of losing weight.

Makes sense, right? Willpower alone would be you telling yourself, "I'll buy the desserts, but I just won't eat them." How well do you think that one will work for you?

What if your goal is too big? Try breaking it down into small (maybe even tiny) steps. For example, if you want to exercise more, start with two push-ups, not fifty. Or if you want to floss your teeth, start with one tooth. Sounds ridiculous, doesn't it? That's actually what it takes to make lasting changes.

Often people feel overwhelmed even with the idea change. How do you fit one more thing into your already packed schedule? Find an anchor. That means that you should anchor the new behavior to an already existing habit. Do you brush your teeth regularly? Then attach flossing to that action. Most people pee an average of seven times a day. What new habit could you attach to that activity? Could you do lunges on your way back to your desk from the bathroom or stretch your arms and legs when you get up from your desk? Sure, you might look silly, but you'd be working out. And who knows, you might even start a new trend at the office.

The big thing to remember is this: if it hurts, you're doing too much. The new behavior needs to not be a big deal.

Remember to acknowledge your successes as well. Look in the mirror and give yourself a thumbs up or a big smile while saying, "Nicely done!" It seems like such a simple thing, yet how often do you celebrate even the tiny successes in your life?

The funny thing about your brain is that it can't distinguish between celebration over something big or something small. By celebrating the small stuff, you leverage that small success into bigger successes. It's a snowball effect. The more small changes you're successful with, the more you increase your confidence and pave the way to reach bigger goals.

As we all know, making changes can be challenging, and without support, you increase your probability of failure. For example, people who are part of a book club tend to read more. People who join an investment club have an easier time figuring out their finances. People who want to be healthier team up with an accountability partner and have regular check-ins. Finding support will not only keep you accountable, but it will motivate you as well. If your friend is waiting for you to show up for that 6:00 a.m. power walk, you won't want to disappoint her. Besides, it's more fun!

Making changes to get healthy can also trigger emotional responses. Many people can be attached to feeling ill or carrying extra weight. When those things begin to shift, they can bring up emotions, such as anxiety, sadness, fear, or anger.

Think about it: when you change your looks or have more energy, you're going to feel different in the world. People around you may treat you differently. Some may like you better overweight and sick. You may attract attention in ways you're not used to. For instance, I'm always amazed when patients make positive changes in their lives that trigger negative reactions from friends and family.

Be aware of this possibility and understand it's not about you; it's triggering fear or some other emotion in them. Take time to check in with yourself as you begin to make shifts and feel better. It's great to have a good friend with whom you can confide. That friend needs to be a good listener and nonjudgmental. A therapist or five-element acupuncturist, because they balance the mind, body, and spirit, could also be a great support person.

Setting Intentions

Intention is in everything. It's important to set your intentions daily and remind yourself of them every day. Here are some examples of daily intention:

Every day and every way, I find ways to be more grateful.
Every day and every way, I find ways to be more outstanding.
I'm happy and healthy.

It's my intention to ...
Live my life with purpose and love
Respect myself and others more often
Create loving relationships
Express my gifts and talents
Feel successful and abundant

Take a minute right now to list five reasons for getting healthy. Look at how your health may influence your spouse, children, or friends.

1.

2.

3.

4.

5.

This list is your *why*. Everyone needs a why. Your why is the reason for doing what you're doing.

Next, look at this list and use it to create one or two simple intentions that you can repeat aloud every day. Put your intentions on a note card and place it where you'll see it several times a day, such as on a bathroom mirror or a nightstand.

Meditation

Did you know that the last thoughts you have before falling asleep will stay in your brain for the next four hours as you sleep? So what are you thinking about before your head hits that pillow and you're off to dream land?

This is one of the reasons I suggest meditating for five minutes before falling asleep. I would also suggest five minutes of meditating upon waking. Who doesn't have five minutes to spare if it would change your life for four hours? (It's one of those one-degree course corrections I mentioned earlier.)

Here are some great reasons to make this small change in your routine:

1. According to a 2014 Johns Hopkins University study. meditation can reduce anxiety and depression,
2. Meditation can improve your attention span in just five days with daily practice.
3. Meditation can improve your mood.
4. Meditation can increase your compassion. We could all use a bit more of this.
5. Meditation can reduce the effects of the stress hormone cortisol. This effect supports a sharper memory, healthier weight, and better sleep.
6. Meditation can slow the aging process by reversing premature aging in cells. (Woohoo!)
7. Meditation can reduce pain.
8. Meditation can support your heart by lowering blood pressure, slowing heart rate, and improving heart health.
9. Meditation helps manage cancer stress symptoms.
10. Meditation can boost your immunity by increasing antibody levels and helping the body fight illnesses and infections.[1]

Meditation can be intimidating for those who have never done it. Maybe you tried it, and it just didn't work for you. My suggestion is that you go into it without expectations. Nothing specific is supposed to happen. It's just about breathing and settling the mind to whatever extent that's possible for you.

Meditation isn't something you do once and then reap major benefits. It's the kind of thing that brings changes over time with small daily effort. If you go to the gym, do a single workout, then go home and look in the mirror, you won't see much difference. Changes to the body don't appear instantly. Yet if you work out over three months and then look at a past photo of yourself, you'll see the change. Meditation is like that. Do it daily, and over time you'll notice that you have started to feel calmer and more balanced.

Current research shows that meditation helps balance the stress response in the body. When stress levels go out of balance, cortisol and adrenaline levels increase. Cortisol and adrenaline are stress hormones that cause a proinflammatory state in the body when they're out of balance. Inflammation is the root cause of degenerative diseases such as Alzheimer's, diabetes, and cancer. Inflammation can also disrupt the digestive system and weaken your immune system.

Daily meditation has been shown to trigger positive cellular and neurological transformations, thereby improving your overall health and happiness. Here's a link that will tell you more about meditation: https://experiencelife.com/article/learning-to-sit-still/.[2]

Practicing regular meditation can decrease physical pain, ease insomnia, increase immunity, lower blood pressure, and relieve the symptoms of many conditions, including irritable bowel syndrome, allergies, asthma, and other chronic illnesses. It's also used in treating depression, anxiety, addiction, and general stress.[3]

So, what have you got to lose?

When you wake up tomorrow morning, sit up in bed, close your eyes, and just breathe deeply for three to five minutes. If thoughts come up about a meeting or you start running through the day's activities, just let your attention notice those thoughts and then let them go. This process is more about quieting the random chatter in our minds (what's known as the "monkey mind") rather than being completely void of thoughts. Let your attention come back to your breath. It's that simple. If you have trouble just breathing and quieting your mind, try just repeating a single word that resonates with you, such as *love* or *peace*.

When you go to bed tonight, follow the same routine. When you finish your five minutes, pause and list a few things that happened today that bring you gratitude. Ask yourself, "What went well for you today?"

I'll expand on this concept in the daily happiness week. For now, just keep it simple.

You'll fall asleep with good thoughts and a clear mind, which will improve the quality of your sleep. Remember, the thoughts you have before bed remain in your subconscious for the next four hours! That is why thoughts of gratitude before sleep are so important. I've heard, "The way you fall asleep is the way you wake up." There's a lot of truth in that saying.

Self-Limiting Beliefs

Brian Tracy says in his book, *Maximum Achievement,* "Your conscious mind can only hold one thought at a time, and you can substitute that one thought for another. This crowding out principle allows you to deliberately replace a negative thought with a positive thought. In so doing, you take control of your emotional life. This law is your key to happiness, to a positive mental attitude, and to personal liberation. It can change your relationships, your conversations, and the predominant content of your conscious mind. Many people have told me thought substitution has changed their lives." [4]

We all have self-limiting beliefs whether we realize it or not. They are the thoughts that poke around in your head, such as "I'm not good enough," "I'm too fat," "I'm lazy," "It's all my fault," and so forth. You know what I'm talking about.

This week is your opportunity to practice more awareness around your thoughts and to start to identify your common limiting beliefs. Start to pay attention to your self-talk. When you hear a limiting belief, take a moment to write it down. Keep a list of the recurring negative thoughts that you tell yourself. This activity will raise your awareness, as you may not even realize how many times you limit yourself in your thoughts.

Next, take that list of self-limiting beliefs and turn them around into positive statements. For example, "I hate exercise" can become "I'm enjoying exercise more." "I'm too fat" can become "I appreciate my health," "I like my eyes," or "My hair is glossy." "I'm so stupid" can become "I can figure things out," "I like my cooking, "I enjoy art," "I'm good at dance," and so forth.

Negative thoughts can become automatic to you. Keep your list of new positive statements handy, as you'll see how to use them in the next section.

How to Stop the Self-Limiting Belief Loop

When you catch yourself in a downward spiral of self-limiting thoughts, just stop. Literally tell yourself "Stop!" Then take a breath and find a turn-around thought to substitute for the self-limiting one. Awareness is the first step, then stopping the action, and then substituting. This will take time and practice. It's not something that changes instantly. Just keep at it, and over time you'll start to notice that you have more positive beliefs than self-limiting ones floating around in your consciousness.

Jill Bolte Taylor, Ph.D., a brain researcher who suffered a stroke, offered these insights into the relationship between thoughts, emotions, and our physical bodies. Hers is an amazing story, and I love her insights.

Emotions release a chemical component in the body that lasts only 90 seconds. At that point, the chemicals have dissipated from your blood and your automatic response is over. If you remain in that emotion, for example, anger, then you are choosing to continue that response. Moment by moment you have the choice to continue along that path or hook into the present moment. Being in the moment will allow that feeling to dissolve. When someone approaches you with anger, you have the choice either to reflect that anger or to approach them with a compassionate heart. What most of us don't realize is that we are unconsciously making choices about how we respond all the time. It is so easy to get caught up in the wiring of our pre-programmed reactivity that we live our lives cruising along on automatic pilot. With this realization, you don't have to think thoughts that bring you pain. There is nothing wrong with thinking about things that bring pain, but it's important to know that you are choosing to go down that thought path. Forgiving others and forgiving yourself is always a choice. Seeing this moment as a perfect moment is always a choice.

The first step to getting out of the negative loop is to recognize when you are in those loops. This takes observation of what your brain is telling you. This will take effort. Learning to listen to your brain from a non-judgmental position may take some practice and patience. This will free you from the worrisome drama of your internal story-teller. Fear, anger, or anxiety can be triggered by all sorts of stimulation. When you are in a negative loop, stop and check in with your body. How is your breathing? Is your stomach upset? These feelings will trigger a physiological response that you can train yourself to notice when it starts. Give yourself 90 seconds for the physiological response to run its course and then gently speak to your brain. Appreciate your ability to think thoughts and then tell your brain that you are no longer interested in thinking these thoughts and feeling these connected emotions. Tell it, "Please stop bringing this stuff up."

This is a conscious effort to stop your brain from hooking into negative thought patterns. You may find a different way to speak to your brain and stop the loop. Try it and see what works best for you. If you are having trouble, you might want to add a kinesthetic trigger such a wiggling a particular finger. Once you have stopped the negative loop, you can then substitute the negative thoughts with something that brings you joy or happiness. Here is where you use your list of thought substitutions that you wrote in the previous section. Think of something in your life that brings you extreme joy and use that as your replacement thought. You must be willing to tend the garden of your mind and make that decision a thousand times a day. [5]

Action Items:

1. Set your intentions; read them aloud daily.
2. Meditate five minutes, two times a day.
3. Substitute limiting beliefs: write, substitute, practice
4. Keep a food log (see format below)

Daily Intake Journal

What did you eat today?

Breakfast _____
_____

Lunch _____
_____

Dinner _____
_____

Other _____
_____

How are you feeling?

Did you experience any physical effects after a meal or snack?

How did you sleep last night?

What exercise did you do today?

Weekly Check-in

At the end of each week, take a moment to reflect and check in with your mind, body, and spirit. How are you feeling in each of these areas?

Rate any of the items listed below that you may be experiencing.

1=very slightly, 2=mild, 3=frequently, and 4=constantly

Add your ratings and make note of the total.

Head
- Headaches
- Dizziness
- Brain fog
- Puffy eyes

Nose
- Nasal congestion
- Excessive mucus
- Stuffy/runny nose
- Clear throat frequently

Lungs and skin
- Chest congestion
- Asthma or bronchitis
- Acne
- Hives, eczema, dry skin
- Excessive sweating

Emotions
- Food cravings
- Emotional eating
- Compulsive eating
- Mood swings
- Depression
- Anxiety
- Nervousness
- Irritability/short temper

Digestion
- Nausea/vomiting
- Diarrhea
- Constipation
- Bloating
- Belching/passing gas
- Heartburn/indigestion
- Intestinal/stomach pain
- Water retention/swelling

Energy
- ○ Fatigue
- ○ Lethargy
- ○ Hyperactivity
- ○ Restlessness
- ○ Sleep quality

Muscles/joints
- ○ Pain/aching joints
- ○ Arthritis
- ○ Muscle stiffness
- ○ Muscle aches
- ○ Weak muscles

TOTAL:

****

[1] Experience Life Staff, "Brain-Body Benefits of Meditation," *Experience Life* (January/February 2015), https//experiencelife.com.

[2] Patrick Downes, "Learning to Sit Still," *Experience Life* (December 2007), https://experiencelife.com.

[3] Patty Onderko, "Meditation-Your Way," *Success Magazine* (May 2014): 36–37.

[4] Brian Tracy,. *Maximum Achievement* (New York: Simon and Schuster Paperbacks, 1993).

[5] Jill Bolte Taylor, *My Stroke of Insight* (London: Viking, 2008).

Week 2

Clean Out Your Pantry and Make a Plan

Week 2 is all about cleaning out your pantry and making a plan. This means a plan for what you are going to eat during the week and writing up your shopping list. I suggest you start with a clean-out of your pantry as detailed below. Then review the fourteen-day meal plan and decide what you'd like to cook this week.

Ask yourself these questions: When is a good day for you to shop? When is a good day to prep the meals for the week? Make a plan to set yourself up for success. If you just go to the store without a plan, food can easily go to waste or prepping a meal may be too much effort after a long day of work.

I like shopping on Fridays and prepping food on Saturdays or Sundays. Write your meal plan on a calendar so that you don't have to think when you're tired and hungry. That's the worst possible time to try to make a food decision. Don't snack while cooking, as those calories can add up pretty darn quickly. Take time to chop and wash veggies. Start with planning meals that take thirty minutes or less. This should be a snap if all the veggies are prewashed and cut.

The Pantry

Start by sorting out what you already have in your pantry. You'll need to schedule at least thirty minutes to get this done. Once you've done the initial clean-out, it will just be a matter of keeping it filled with healthy, low-glycemic options.

Start by emptying everything onto the counter. Read the labels of cereals, crackers, and any other processed foods you may have around. As a general rule, look for foods that are twenty-three carbs per serving or less. These are foods that won't spike your blood sugar levels. You'll be surprised at how many carbs per serving most packaged goods contain.

Toss out all high-glycemic processed foods like crackers, bread, pasta, chips, cookies, sugar, syrups, and so forth Also toss all expired or suspicious foods (e.g., old cracker boxes, ancient bags of flour, outdated canned goods). Toss out old dried herbs and ground spices, as these should be replaced every six months.

Take a damp sponge and wipe down all the shelves. Take time to remove honey and jam stickiness. You want to start fresh, and having a clean pantry is a great place to start. Reload the pantry. Put everyday stuff like USANA's My Smart Food shakes and bars, and low-glycemic snacks at the most accessible levels. Organize items into logical groups such as baking supplies, canned goods, and so forth. Store oils like olive and sesame in the fridge, as they do go rancid. I keep a small container of olive oil on the counter so that it is handy for cooking. Each week I refill it. Also, get rid of corn and canola oil unless they are organic, as they are genetically modified organisms (GMO) otherwise.

Clean Your Brain

Now that you've cleaned out your pantry, it's time to tackle your brain. I love what Darren Hardy says about how what you put in your face is the result you get. He is talking not only about food but media.

What do you watch and read on a regular basis? This is where I want to suggest that you reduce your exposure to toxic media.

What other kind of media is out there? There are constant messages in the media that tell you that you need to be thinner, richer, more beautiful, more fearful, and so forth. What you put in your mind is what you will think about. So my suggestion for you is that for the next seven days, stop reading the news and watching the news and any television. Give your brain a detox. You'll actually be amazed as to how much "extra" time you'll have to do things you've really wanted to do.

I've done this and never turned back. After spending a month in India studying yoga with BKS Iyengar, I came back and didn't resume my nightly TV watching. I used to eat dinner and then watch an hour or so of TV. I grew up with a single mom who worked two jobs to support us. That meant I had free rein watching TV. After not watching TV for an entire month while in India, I realized I didn't really miss it. Now, don't get me wrong, I do watch a show here and there and do love movies, but it's no longer a daily habit.

I also used to be a news junkie. I listened to National Public Radio (NPR) almost 24/7. I worked in the environmental field, and I stayed on top of every horrible thing that was happening in the world. Then, I decided to take a break from the daily onslaught of negativity. And, you know what happened? I didn't miss it and I realized I didn't need to know everything. What I did instead was began reading positive media such as *Success Magazine*, which focuses on what people are doing in the world to make a difference. I also visit http://www.happify.com to watch inspirational videos.

Many people fear that they will miss something important if they don't watch TV news, read newspapers, or listen to news radio. Believe me, you will find out about something important if you need to know about it. When my mom starts a sentence with "Did you see in the news what happened to those children?" I say, "Stop. Is this something I really need to know about or will it just be a sad, horrible story?" I can't recall once where she completed the story. Now she has reduced her daily news intake and no longer shares negative stories with me. I am a lot happier in my daily life without starting the day with the barrage of negativity. Give it a try. I think you'll love it too.

Make a Meal Plan

Next, it's time to make a plan. Most people resist food planning, complaining that it's too time consuming. I assure you, once you get into the habit of planning, it will be a breeze. It may even become fun! I encourage you to consider how simple it is to plan and eat a healthy menu that does not spike your blood sugar.

Remember to start with a simple step. Go to the Resources Section of this workbook and pick out some meals you'd like to try. You don't have to plan all fourteen days of meals in the next two weeks. How about planning just three meals this week or planning snacks for the week? Begin with small changes, and once you've implemented those, they will lead to bigger changes. If you never shop with a list, start there. Plan one meal and some snacks and just shop for those ingredients. This is how you make long-term changes.

So here's the basic outline of how to eat. It's not rocket science, and it's nothing you haven't heard before. I am going to encourage you to eliminate all breads, grains, cereals, rice, pasta, potatoes, sugar, candy, soda, and fruit juices for at least one to two weeks. You will reintroduce some of these foods, but they will be breads, rice, cereals, and potatoes that will not spike your blood sugar. Remember not to go hungry; however, if you do eat an additional meal or snack, I want it to be a meal or snack that does not spike your blood sugar; so think protein with a veggie or fruit.

Start your day with warm lemon water. Why? This helps with digestion and increases hydrochloric acid (HCL). HCL decreases with age and stress. The water also hydrates you after eight hours of sleep. Yes, I said eight hours! More on that later in this book.

Eat breakfast with some protein. Studies have shown that those who eat a breakfast with some protein were found to eat 80 percent fewer calories throughout the day. Have you ever thought to yourself that you'd just skip breakfast to lose a little weight only to find yourself eating continuously from dinner to bedtime? That's the problem. Don't ever skip a meal. Decide instead to eat about every four hours. It's very important to eat within one hour of rising so your blood sugar levels don't plummet in the morning. Eat dinner between 5 p.m. and 7 p.m. for proper digestion and to have a couple of hours before bed to digest your food. Stop all food and water intake by 8pm.

Action Items:

1. Clean out your pantry.
2. Clean your brain with a media diet.
3. Plan your meals.
4. Start your day with lemon water.
5. Eat within one hour of rising.
6. Eat protein with every meal.
7. Eat every four hours.
8. Never skip a meal.

Daily Intake Journal

What did you eat today?

Breakfast _____

_____

Lunch _____

_____

Dinner _____

_____

Other _____

_____

How are you feeling?

Did you experience any physical effects after a meal or snack?

How did you sleep last night?

What exercise did you do today?

Weekly Check-in

At the end of each week, take a moment to reflect and check in with your mind, body, and spirit. How are you feeling in each of these areas?

Rate any of the items listed below that you may be experiencing.

1=very slightly, 2=mild, 3=frequently, and 4=constantly

Add your ratings and make note of the total.

Head
- Headaches
- Dizziness
- Brain fog
- Puffy eyes

Nose
- Nasal congestion
- Excessive mucus
- Stuffy/runny nose
- Clear throat frequently

Lungs and skin
- Chest congestion
- Asthma or bronchitis
- Acne
- Hives, eczema, dry skin
- Excessive sweating

Emotions
- o Food cravings
- o Emotional eating
- o Compulsive eating
- o Mood swings
- o Depression
- o Anxiety
- o Nervousness
- o Irritability/short temper

Digestion
- o Nausea/vomiting
- o Diarrhea
- o Constipation
- o Bloating
- o Belching/passing gas
- o Heartburn/indigestion
- o Intestinal/stomach pain
- o Water retention/swelling

Energy
- o Fatigue
- o Lethargy
- o Hyperactivity
- o Restlessness
- o Sleep quality

Muscles/joints
- o Pain/aching joints
- o Arthritis
- o Muscle stiffness
- o Muscle aches
- o Weak muscles

TOTAL:

WEEK 3

Supplements and Skin Care

What's the Cheapest Health Insurance?

(Thanks to Dr. Myron Wentz for his 2014 presentation, which inspired this section of my workbook.) [1]

Did you know that people who lack vitamin D have twice the risk of developing Alzheimer's disease? We need vitamin supplementation more today than ever before. Our environment is unfriendly to our health. However, the correct nutrients in the proper amounts can protect you from degenerative diseases. The problem is that all our nutrition comes from our food, and our food no longer contains the levels of nutrients our body needs for optimal health.

Problems start on the farm with fertilizers and monoculture. There is far too little concern for the health of the soil. Our nutrient-rich topsoil is depleting 100 times faster than it can regenerate.

We need forty different nutrients in our body to be healthy. Fruits and vegetables, which are picked before they're fully mature in order to be shipped and stored, lack nutrients. The storing of food increases the loss of nutrients. Processing foods take out the nutrients. Our soil is depleted of nutrients as well.

The Average White Potato Has Lost 100% of Its Vitamin A!

Our reliance on genetically modified crops is leading to greater application of herbicides and other chemicals. Chemicals and toxins in our food and environment force our bodies to cope. Cord blood was tested in newborn U.S. babies and showed 287 toxic chemicals in the blood. Children are being born with toxins that their little bodies have to work to clear out. Some of the chemicals found in their blood were ones that have been banned for over thirty years. This shows us that there are some toxins that our bodies just can't clear out. No longer will just a healthy diet will work for us. Our bodies need more protection and nourishment even before birth.

Modern technologies expose us to drugs that keep our bodies from absorbing nutrients. Statin drugs stop the body from absorbing CoQ10, for example. Antidepressants deplete the body of nutrients, and once the body is depleted, the drug becomes less effective. That's when doctors prescribe new drugs, and the depletion continues.

* Check out Drug muggers in the resources section to see the full list of pharmaceutical drugs and the nutrients they deplete from the body.

Poor nutrition is often the result of poor food choices. Convenience and taste ranked higher than health in studies about what kids like for lunch. Did you know a child's palate (their taste preferences) is set by the age of five? That means if a child's diet consists of processed food from an early age, the child will develop a taste preference for those foods, causing whole food choices to be unappealing. That's why it's essential to introduce your child to a variety of whole foods from the very start.

No Longer Will a Healthy Diet Be Enough to Keep Us Healthy

Thousands of studies prove the benefits of taking micronutrients. The need for optimal health is evident. The cheapest health insurance is a high-quality, pharmaceutical-grade nutritional supplement. It's the most cost effective health insurance practice.

Four Main Reasons You Are Nutrient-Depleted
from Dr. Mark Hyman

There are numerous reasons most of us are nutrient malnourished, anything from eroding topsoil depleting our mineral supply, to a toxic environment and the abundance of junk food many Americans eat. If I had to narrow nutrient depletion down to four primary reasons, this is what I would say:

1. We evolved eating wild foods that contained dramatically higher levels of all vitamins, minerals, and essential fats.

2. Because of depleted soils, industrial farming and hybridization techniques, the animals and vegetables we eat have fewer nutrients.

3. Processed factory-made foods have no nutrients.

4. The total burden of environmental toxins, lack of sunlight and chronic stress lead to higher nutrient needs.

These are among the reasons why everyone, at the very least, needs a good multivitamin, fish oil and vitamin D. I also recommend probiotics because modern life, diet and antibiotics, as well as other drugs, damage our gut ecosystem, which is so important in keeping us healthy and thin.[2]

I often hear patients say they don't believe in vitamins, and they just eat healthily and feel that's sufficient.

Well, that's what I used to think until I looked at the research and started taking a high-quality supplement. After just one week, I actually felt the difference.

1. Current science shows that it takes eight oranges today to equal the vitamin C content found in one orange from 1900.
2. To get the iron you would have eaten in one cup of spinach in 1945, you'd have to eat sixty-four cups today.

3. Even the American Medical Association suggests supplements!
4. Be aware! Not all supplements are the same. Some contain contaminants like mercury, lead, and cheap fillers that inhibit or block absorption.

I had a client who wanted to lose weight before getting pregnant with her second child. Although that was her ultimate goal, what she really shifted when she started my supplement protocol were her general health and well-being. As her health and well-being improved, she was able to reduce her weight naturally and then easily get pregnant as a result of her healthier body.

How to Select a Good Vitamin and Mineral Supplement

1. **Is the supplement safe to take?**

   Multi-vitamin supplements are a combination of ingredients and can contain substances that are not listed on the label. Science-based nutrition companies will test ingredients for contaminants such as E. coli, salmonella, pesticides, steroids, stimulants, and other banned substances. In addition, vitamins and minerals can contain toxic levels from inconsistencies in the strength of raw materials. Make sure the nutrition company tests every batch of pills to confirm that the strength and purity are consistent and safe.

2. **Am I getting what's on the label?**

   To insure that what's on the label (and only what's on the label) is in the bottle, only buy products that adhere to Pharmaceutical Good Manufacturing Process (GMP). These are the rigorous standards that govern the production of prescription and over-the-counter medications. Most vitamins are manufactured under FDA guidelines only, *which do not ensure that what is on the label is in the bottle.*

3. Does the supplement get absorbed?

A multi-vitamin or mineral is only as good as its ability to be absorbed and utilized in the body. It is important to choose supplements that meet U.S. Pharmacopeia standards for disintegration and dissolution. Look for a supplement with chelated minerals in it, so you can be sure that your body will absorb them. Also, be sure that there is an expiration date indicating when the supplement may no longer meet United States Pharmacopeia (USP) standards of quality and strength.

4. Is the company science-based and credible?

Is the company research-based and science-focused? Who is the formulator of the products? Do you know that by ordering as few as 100 bottles, anyone can have their own vitamin brand? Just a few manufacturers produce most of the vitamins sold to several thousand companies. Look for a company that manufacturers their own products. Look for a company that is tested and certified by independent agencies such as NSF International, Consumer Labs or Nutrisearch Inc.

Printed with permission from Pamela J. Firle, M.A., L.P.C. (http://wholehealthwise.com/wp-content/uploads/2012/10/ How-to-Select-a-Good-Vitamin-and-Mineral-Supplement.pdf)

I use The Nutrisearch Comparative Guide to Nutritional Supplements by Lyle MacWilliam for a third-party analysis of over 1500 products on 18 different criteria available in the U.S. and Canada. [3]

Manufacturing Excellence: The Building Blocks of a Better Supplement

I'd like to share with you why I believe USANA supplements are the best. My whole family takes them, and we love them. I've used them with my patients as well. Many people take poor quality supplements and don't even realize how poor they are. If you are taking a supplement and want to know the quality, I'll be happy to look up their rating in my reference book.

USANA Health Sciences is the manufacturer of the supplements I recommend and trust with my family. USANA manufactures excellence in their product line. They only source the highest quality raw materials for their supplements. If it doesn't meet their high standards, they won't use it. For example, grape seed extract, to most people, is just something extracted from a grape seed. "To scientists in the labs of USANA Health Sciences, grape seed extract is a complex mixture of organic compounds containing 80–90 percent phenols (also known as proanthocyanidins) and 10–15 percent monomer content. They have seen bad samples from prospective suppliers that contain less than five percent phenols and no monomers. The material USANA purchases is on the high end of the price spectrum, but it's well worth it because the extract contains greater than 80 percent phenols and has monomer content of about 10 or 15 percent. USANA has been using the product for almost 20 years now, with great results."[4]

I trust that USANA does a superior job in choosing the highest quality raw materials and testing them to assure quality to make the #1 rated (by Nutrisearch) nutritional supplement in North America.

As of August 2016, USANA has gone beyond what any other nutritional supplement company has to offer and reformulated their supplements with cell signaling technology.

USANA's new InCelligence Technology uses nutrients and plant-derived biomolecules to target specific cell-signaling pathways that
1. Unlock the code of your innate cellular intelligence
2. Trigger your body's natural protection and renewal mechanisms
3. Build your cellular resistance (the ability of your cells to adapt to stress)
4. Change USANA's approach to formulating new products

CellSentials is formulated with InCelligence cell-signaling technology to unlock vibrant health. The powerful combination of Core Minerals and Vita-Antioxidant supplements provides the triple-action support your body needs to nourish, protect, and renew your cells.

There are other products that claim to use cell signaling. But they only target one cellular communication pathway with a limited number of nutrients. InCelligence takes a broader approach. Using a blend of powerful nutrients to signal more processes, USANA created the most effective, holistic approach to your health.

The secret of Beautiful Skin

What is the best way to have younger, healthier, more vibrant skin? There are so many options out there, confusion and overwhelm can take over your brain in the beauty isle. It's just too hard to know what to do. What type of skin calls for which kind of product? What are truly safe ingredients?

When we get older, our skin starts to sag and loses its radiance. We look in the mirror and see the crow's feet, dull/dry skin, sagging under our arms (isn't that one a favorite?).

What we really would like instead is smooth, glowing skin.

When you take a high quality nutritional supplement, it works from the inside out. It will make your skin more radiant and glowing. When you use high quality skin care products they will work at a cellular level to make your skin look and feel younger.

I'd like to share a true story. I had this guy taking the USANA supplements to help his overall health and specifically his joint pain. He felt better overall and had less joint pain after taking the supplements for a few months. The next time I saw him, he asked me, "do these supplements make you look younger?" I told him they can, because they work from the inside out at the DNA level. He then said, "because people keep asking me what I'm doing because I am looking younger!"

When you think about your skin, it's more about what you put into your mouth rather than what you put on your skin that makes a difference. Your skin reflects what is going on inside your body. Skin is the body's largest organ. Don't get me wrong, high quality, preservative free skin care is essential, but I want to share with you a few tips on what can help from the inside out.

There are 3 layers of skin. The outside layer (epidermis) is made up of dead skin cells that have migrated to the surface from the inner layers. Once those cells are exposed to the air, they die. That's good because it provides protection for your body. This process happens every 28 days. So, if you take care of what's going on inside your body, you'll see the changes on your skin in just 4-8 weeks.

The middle layer (dermis) is like a great big sponge that hydrates your skin. So, my first tip is to DRINK WATER and plenty of it. How much water is good? Well, if you weigh 100 pounds, then shoot for 50oz of water per day. So that's about half your body weight in ounces. The easiest way to start is by beginning your day with warm lemon water as that will hydrate you and also help aid in digestion. Good digestion is key to good skin.

The bottom layer (subcutaneous) is where cellulite, which is bands of fat, get trapped and hangout. To make a difference in that layer you need to stimulate the lymphatic system. The lymph glands move the waste of the body to your liver to be detoxed and then eliminated by the kidneys. To help move lymph, I suggest a Chi machine. It's relatively inexpensive and can be ordered on Amazon. What is does is move the body in a slight back and forth motion thereby stimulating the lymph to drain. I find it quite relaxing and do it every night before bed and use it as a time to meditate and release everything from the day.

You have the power to make a difference in your skin by aiding your skin's natural ability to eliminate toxins. When the elimination systems of the body, the liver, kidneys, and digestion, are not working properly, then the toxins come out on the skin as acne, for example. If the acne is on the chin, it's related to digestion problems. Around the jaw line relates to sex hormone imbalances.

Stress can wreak havoc on your skin. Living in an amped up adrenaline state, the fight or flight hormone, whacks out your body's ability to function normally. Adrenaline communicates to every cell in the body that you are in danger even though that danger may be just an inbox full of emails. Your heart rate increases, your blood pressure goes up and your pupils dilate because the body thinks it's in danger.

When you are in a state of stress response, the blood flow gets diverted away from digestion to your arms and legs so that you can run from danger. Since you don't run from your emails, or maybe some of you do, the adrenaline just keeps pumping out. Digestion slows down as a result and you start to see acne on the face or you'll have dry, brittle hair and nails because the nutrients are being diverted elsewhere to save your life.

Focus on optimizing digestion to improve your skin. When living with stress, you need to add restorative processes in your life, like deep breathing. Deep, diaphragmatic breathing actually stimulates the parasympathetic nervous system and calms everything down. This tells your body that everything is ok, and you are not in danger.

Eat Fat. Yes, I really mean it and it won't make you fat. It's a wonderful fuel that nourishes the skin and reduces inflammation that causes aging. Our body does not produce fatty acids so they have to be consumed. There are 2 types, omega 3's and omega 6's. Most people get too many of the omega 6's. Examples are poultry, eggs, cereals, wheat, most veggie oils, corn oil, safflower oil, and coconut to name a few. Omega 3's are anti-inflammatory. They nourish the skin and increase softness and decreases wrinkles. Examples of omega 3's are flax seeds and oil, chia seeds, walnuts, pecans and oily fish. USANA has a clean and safe fish oil supplement that contains lemon oil so you don't burp fish! Eat avocados. They are a great source of fat and have 19 different vitamins and minerals. They are a "good" fat.

Omega 3's are incorporated into the outside layer of every cell in the body. It keeps cells flexible and it drives the anti-inflammation process, which literally slows down the aging process from the inside out.

Signs of deficiency include cracked elbows, cracked heels or generally dry skin. Focus on getting more omega 3's into your daily diet.

Vitamin C. We know it's good for colds, but how does it help your skin? It increases circulation, which helps you grow healthier hair. It makes collagen and elastin, which help tendons and ligaments repair and stay healthy. So this is essential for people who work out or do sports.

Vitamin C decreases free radical damage. As you breathe, you take in oxygen and expel carbon dioxide. That leaves a single oxygen molecule roaming around your body and that generates something called free radicals. Antioxidants donate a single oxygen molecule, the two pair up and damage stops. You also get oxidative stress with sun exposure and pollution. Those free radicals consume collagen and fibrinogen causing wrinkles and aging.

Some signs of vitamin C deficiency are premature aging, broken capillaries, easy bruising, hair breaking easily, and hair loss. Some natural sources are berries, kale, and parsley. It's also essential to take a pharmaceutical grade nutritional supplement that has optimal levels of antioxidants.

Dark circles. You get 8 hours of sleep and yet you still wake with those dark circles that make you look like you've been out partying all night. What causes those dark circles under eyes? They reflect what is going on in the elimination and detoxing systems of the body. The liver and kidneys are the main organs involved. To support the digestion process, decrease or eliminate the following:
Alcohol, more than 5 drinks per week increases oxidative damage
Caffeine
Sugar
Gluten, not easily digested
Casein, in dairy products

Sleep! It's essential to your health and beauty. Get 7-9 hours of sleep a night. It's also important that those hours begin by 10pm. In Chinese medicine, as well as western clinical studies, it has been found that sleep in the earlier part of the night rejuvenates and replenishes the body more effectively than going to bed later and sleeping the same amount of hours. Create a bedtime ritual where an hour before your bedtime, turn down the lights, turn off the electronics and do things that are relaxing. If you like to read in bed, read from an old school real book, no electronic devices. Don't sleep with any electronics in the bedroom. Get one of those old-fashioned battery operated alarm clocks so there is no light in the room while you sleep.

Not only do I recommend USANA Health Sciences brand of supplements to all my patients, but I also recommend the USANA skin care line, Sensé. The skin care line is completely free of all preservatives and has a unique self-preserving system. Did you know that what you put on your skin, can be found in your blood stream within twenty minutes? So it's super important to pay attention to what is in your skin care products.

I used to have dry skin and tried all types of products to get it looking better, but nothing ever really worked and I spent a ton of money on those products. Once I started taking the supplements and using the skin care line, which was less expensive than the others, my skin balanced out and is now no longer dry.

Take a minute now and look at the products you are currently using. Do they have any of the following chemicals? If they do, toss them out immediately.

1. **Artificial Fragrances aka Phthalates** (like benzene and toluene)— these are hormone disruptors.
2. **Sodium Lauryl and Sodium Laureth Sulfate** (SLS)— These make things lather. They are hormone disruptors and carcinogenic.
3. **Butylated Hydroxyanisole** (BHA)— A common preservative. It's carcinogenic and has been shown to cause thyroid and reproductive issues.
4. **Parabens**—These are very common preservative. They disrupt hormones, can cause reproductive issues, and linked to higher incidence of breast cancer.

5. **Polyethylene Glycol** (PEG)—This is a powerful de-greaser and used in oven cleaners. It actually shows up in baby wipes, cleansers, lip balm, and lotions. It's been linked with kidney damage and several types of cancers.

Invest in taking care of your skin from the inside and you'll see wonderful results on the outside.

Action Items:

1. Start taking high quality nutritional supplements (contact me if you want USANA).
2. If you currently take supplements, find out the quality rating.
3. Keep up on your food log.
4. Clean out all your bath and body products.
5. Fill out your weekly reflections chart.
6. Plan five meals this week.

Daily Intake Journal

What did you eat today?

Breakfast _____

_____

Lunch _____

_____

Dinner _____

_____

Other _____

_____

How are you feeling?

Did you experience any physical effects after a meal or snack?

How did you sleep last night?

What exercise did you do today?

Weekly Check-in

At the end of each week, take a moment to reflect and check in with your mind, body, and spirit. How are you feeling in each of these areas?

Rate any of the items listed below that you may be experiencing.

1=very slightly, 2=mild, 3=frequently, and 4=constantly

Add your ratings and make note of the total.

Head
- Headaches
- Dizziness
- Brain fog
- Puffy eyes

Nose
- Nasal congestion
- Excessive mucus
- Stuffy/runny nose
- Clear throat frequently

Lungs and skin
- Chest congestion
- Asthma or bronchitis
- Acne
- Hives, eczema, dry skin
- Excessive sweating

Emotions
- Food cravings
- Emotional eating
- Compulsive eating
- Mood swings
- Depression
- Anxiety
- Nervousness
- Irritability/short temper

Digestion
- Nausea/vomiting
- Diarrhea
- Constipation
- Bloating
- Belching/passing gas
- Heartburn/indigestion
- Intestinal/stomach pain
- Water retention/swelling

Energy
- Fatigue
- Lethargy
- Hyperactivity
- Restlessness
- Sleep quality

Muscles/joints
- Pain/aching joints
- Arthritis
- Muscle stiffness
- Muscle aches
- Weak muscles

TOTAL:

****

[1] Myron Wentz, "Optimal Nutrition Is by Far the Most Important Thing You can Do Towards Good Health" (March 2014), http://dbsenterprises.usana.com.

[2] Mark Hyman, "Why You Need to Take Supplements", *EcoWatch* (May 6, 2015), http://ecowatch.com/2015/05/06/dr-hyman-take-supplements.

[3] Lyle MacWilliam, *The Nutrisearch Comparative Guide to Nutritional Supplements,* Northern Dimensions, Vernon, British Columbia, Canada. 2007.

[4] David Baker, "Manufacturing Excellence: The Building Blocks of a Better Supplement," *USANA Health Science,* https://www.usana.com/dotCom/about/MANEXRawMaterials2.

WEEK 4

Digestion

You've heard it a million times: drink water. But how much? A good target amount to drink is about half your body weight in ounces of water. So if you weigh a hundred pounds you would drink fifty ounces of water. Drinking water increases your metabolism by three percent. So when you think you're hungry, drink water first. Thirst and hunger can often be confused.

Start your day with warm lemon water, and add one glass of water after eating. If you link eating and drinking water, then you are more likely to start and retain the new habit. Remember this from Week 1? Link a newly desired habit with an existing one and voilà! You'll have a new habit that will stick.

Your Digestion

Most people think their digestion is perfectly fine and don't realize all the signs and symptoms that can actually point to poor digestion. I have a friend who passes gas very loudly after every meal. He believes this to be normal and refuses to consider that eating does not need to cause excessive gas. Gas and bloating are just a couple of signs your digestion is off track.

The digestive system is made up of a long tube and includes numerous organs including the liver, gallbladder, and pancreas. Each organ has a specific function in digesting food. Without proper digestion, you won't be able to absorb the nutrients from the food you are eating or the vitamins you are taking. Amazingly, 60–70 percent of your immune system is located in the mucosal lining of the GI tract, and 85 percent of your serotonin (happiness hormone) is produced there as well.

Digestion begins in the brain. Take a moment right now and close your eyes and imagine eating the most wonderful piece of chocolate. Feel it melt in your mouth and smell the cocoa. Did you start to salivate? Well, that is digestion starting to happen. Your brain registers that food is coming, and your saliva glands start to put out enzymes needed to break down food.

Start your meal by taking three to five deep belly breaths. This will stimulate the parasympathetic nervous system and reduce stress. When you eat in a rushed or frantic way, you'll be in sympathetic system mode, which is on alert for danger and will cause your body to divert resources from the digestive process. Blood will go out to your extremities because it thinks you're going to need to run from the saber-toothed tiger!

The number one tip I have for good digestion is to chew your food thoroughly. That means twenty to thirty chews per bite. I know, you're thinking that's crazy, but give it a try. Slow down. Really smell and taste your food. Put down the fork and knife between bites and *never* put more food in your mouth until you've completely chewed and swallowed the first bite. I find that taking smaller bites helps this process immensely.

When you eat, your body puts out insulin. Insulin is a fat storage hormone. Carbohydrates break down into sugar, and then insulin breaks it down and stores it in muscle. If there is too much, it then gets stored as fat, mostly around your middle, creating the beloved "spare tire" or "muffin top."

Your stomach then gets the signal to start producing hydrochloric acid (HCL), which breaks down proteins. Because your stomach produces less HCL as you age, I suggest using digestive enzymes supplements with every meal.

To aid digestion, drink warm lemon water before meals. Warm lemon water is especially helpful first thing in the morning to help with hydration and elimination. If you must drink liquids while eating, take small sips and consume as little as possible. Liquids during the meal reduce HCL levels and inhibit the digestive process. Stomach acid kills off bad bacteria, so you want it to be high. It will help stave off food poisoning and helps you from getting sick.

Heartburn is thought to be the most common digestive disorder in the United States, affecting 25 million people per day. Many people believe heartburn is caused by too much stomach acid, when quite the opposite is true. Heartburn is a result of too *little* stomach acid, which invites pathogenic bacteria into the gut to cause bacterial overgrowth or infection.

Here are five simple tips that you can use to get rid of heartburn for good:

1. Make sure that you have enough stomach acid for digestion to fight pathogenic bacteria. At first, this may mean taking a hydrochloric acid (HCL) supplement.
2. Reduce your carbohydrate and sugar intake.
3. Increase gut motility. Take a digestive enzyme.
4. Increase friendly bacteria in your gut. Eat fermented foods and take probiotics.
5. Eat an alkaline diet such as beets, broccoli, cabbage, carrot, cauliflower, celery, chard greens, apple, apricot, avocado, banana (high-glycemic), berries, blackberries, and cantaloupe. This is only a short list. To see the full list, go to this link: http://www.rense.com/1.mpicons/acidalka.htm.

The liver produces bile that helps break down fats. Important vitamins found in foods such as dairy are K, E, A, and D. So eat dairy that is *full fat*. Yes, organic, full-fat dairy is the best way to get these vitamins. Remember, fat doesn't make you fat. Eating fat helps you feel fuller as well.

Be aware of your portion sizes. A half to a three-quarters of your plate should be veggies, a fourth lean protein, and a fourth complex carb (like brown rice, quinoa, sweet potato, or squash).

Your stomach has to stretch to accommodate the food you put in it. Once your stomach gets used to being stretched out, it expects it every day, and this stretching is the reason why, if you choose to diet, you tend to feel hungry after your meals for about four days. Get in the habit of eating more slowly, chewing thoroughly, and checking in with yourself when you're 70-80 percent full. Then stop eating. I know firsthand how challenging this can be when the food tastes good.

It's essential to eat some protein at each meal. When you eat proteins and fats, signals get sent to the brain telling it you are eating. These signals usually reach the brain within five minutes of chewing. By including fats and proteins with each meal, you are likely to eat less and be more satisfied.

Once your food leaves the stomach, it goes to the small intestine. The function of the small intestine is to absorb all the vitamins and minerals from your food. Next, your food passes to the large intestine. There are seven to nine pounds of bacteria living in the large intestine! Some are good and some are bad. You want more good than bad. That's why a probiotic is so important. I suggest my patients take them daily. Eating fermented foods like sauerkraut, miso, tempeh, kimchi, or kefir are great sources of probiotics.

It's also important to choose foods that contain natural sugars and fibers to feed those good bacteria. These are called prebiotics. Some great prebiotic foods are asparagus, bananas, garlic, onions, cabbage, beans, artichokes, apples, leeks, and root veggies such as sweet potatoes, carrots, and beets.

If your food is not properly digested before it gets to the large intestine, the break-down process will cause gas and bloating. Sound like anyone you know?

Things that can affect digestion poorly are

- Caffeine
- Alcohol
- Fatty foods
- Soda
- Ice water
- Poor sleep
- Some medications
- Stress

Eat More Fiber

The typical American diet includes too many fast foods and processed foods like chips, crackers, candy, and pastries, which contain very little fiber. The average fiber intake is about 15g per day, while the recommended serving for women is at least 25g and for men, 38g. Most of us are only getting about half of what our body really needs to be healthy.

The gut is the hub of your immune system (70–80 percent) as well as producing about 85 percent of your serotonin (the happiness hormone). Fiber can help to prevent weight gain and digestive problems. It can help lower cholesterol and help to prevent heart disease. It even works to help control blood sugar levels.

To get 30g fiber, you'd have to eat 8 cups of lentils or 7.5 apples or 3 avocados or 5 cups of broccoli or 7.5 cups oatmeal. See the chart below for more ways to increase your daily fiber. You can also add powdered fiber to your smoothie or protein shake. I use USANA's Fibergy, as it contains 12g per serving.

Food	Serving	Carbs (grams)	Fiber (grams)
1. Avocado (raw)	1 medium	17.1	11
2. Artichoke	1 medium	14.3	10.3
3. Raspberries (raw)	1 cup	15	8
4. Blackberries (raw)	1 cup	15	8
5. Lentils	1/2 cup	9.9	7.9
6. Black Beans	1/2 cup	22	7.3
7. Broccoli	1 cup	9	6
8 Soup, Vegetable Beef*	1 cup	22	5
9. Pear (raw)	1 medium	20	4.5
10. Apple (raw)	1 medium	23	4
11. Oatmeal	1 cup	27	4
12. Barley	1/2 cup	22	3
13. Pumpkin	1 cup, mashed	12	2.9
14. Spinach	1 cup	3.5	2.5
15.Eggplant	1/2 slice	8	2.3
16. Summer Squash	1/2 cup	4	1.9
17. Peach (raw)	1 medium	12	1.8
18. Grapefruit (raw)	1/2 cup sections	10	1.5
19. Tofu, Firm	1/5 pkg.	3	1.5
20. Cauliflower	1/2 cup	2.7	1.3
21. Asparagus	4 spears	2.5	1.2
22. Cabbage	1/2 cup, shredded	3.9	1.2
23. Popcorn	1 cup	6.1	1.2
24. Arugula (raw)	1 cup	2.9	1
25. Olives*	10 olives	1	1

In addition to adding fiber, I suggest all my patients take a liver supporting supplement. A healthy, functioning liver is important to digestion. When we consume alcohol, prescriptions drugs, cigarettes, or caffeine, these substances block the liver, which is the body's detoxification organ. Cholesterol is processed by the liver, so when the liver is already overloaded, the cholesterol is circulated back into the blood stream. This is can cause people have high cholesterol. I like USANA's Hepasil DTX as it contains milk thistle extract to help stimulate enzymes in the liver and contains antioxidants like green tea extract and turmeric to protect against oxidative stress.

Poor digestion can lead to other diseases in the body such as Crohn's disease, irritable bowel syndrome (IBS), diabetes, fibromyalgia, rheumatoid arthritis, restless leg syndrome, and acne.

Start supporting your digestion by removing harmful foods from your diet (like GMOs), reduce stress, eat foods high in antioxidants, take probiotics and quality nutritional supplements, get better sleep, be cautious with antibiotics, and move your body daily.

Remove Toxins From Your Diet

Using USANA's Essentials (a multivitamin) and Hepasil DTX (liver support) will ensure that inflammation is reduced and detoxification is enhanced. Toxins damage cell membranes and block hormone receptor sites that are responsible for assisting with fat loss. Toxins damage the energy-producing (fat-burning) aspects of the cell. Additionally, toxins create more oxidative stress in your body. This leads to slower fat loss and the dreaded premature aging!

Saccharine is carcinogenic. Aspartame is toxic to the brain, is addictive, and also desensitizes the tongue to sugar so that it takes more sugar to make something taste sweet. Studies have shown that diet sodas sweetened with aspartame actually cause weight gain. Sucralose is made by adding chlorine to glucose. Chlorinated glucose, or more commonly known as Splenda, mimics iodine and disrupts normal thyroid function. Take all of these out of your diet immediately. The other brand names of these chemical substitutes for sugar are Sweet'N Low and NutraSweet.[1]

Diet sodas trick your brain so that it wants to consume more calories. Sodas contain a lot of sodium that just makes your thirstier. If you enjoy soda, try substituting mineral water with a splash of real fruit juice or a couple of drops of flavored stevia. Whatever you do, stop drinking soda, especially diet ones.

Wheat produced in the United States currently contains 90 percent more gluten than it did two generations ago. It also contains a protein that suppresses your brain signals that alert you when you are full. People are eating an average of 440 more calories per day. Scary! For more details check out the book *Wheat Belly: Lose the Wheat, Lose the Weight, and Find Your Path Back to Health* by William Davis.

I'm sure you've heard even more stories about toxic ingredients in processed foods. The bottom line is, eliminate them from your diet. They are *not* real food that will nourish you in any way.

Fluoride

Since about 1945, fluoride has been added to many water supplies in the United States. The original thought was that consuming this substance would help prevent cavities in children under the age of six. But in actuality there are several health problems that result from consuming fluoride. From lower fertility rates to thyroid function disruption and neurological effects, fluoride is a toxic element that you need to reduce your exposure to. A study requested by the EPA and recently issued by the National Research Council reported that "high levels of fluoride that occur naturally in some drinking water can cause tooth and bone damage, and should be reduced." [2]

Many studies have shown the affects of fluoride on bones and teeth. Fluoride is helpful in small amounts, but over a certain threshold the affects become negative, resulting in weaker, more brittle bones. At higher concentrations, fluoride is toxic. Moderate to high fluoride exposure in children may result in dental fluorosis. Fluorosis begins with small, white striations across teeth, but it can progress to discolored, pitted teeth that are subject to fracture. [3]

The chemicals used to artificially fluoridate the water supply are actually the waste products from phosphate mining and manufacturing. This means the fertilizer industry gets to offload its toxic waste to water districts around the country and do so as a public health product![4]

You get fluoride in your tap water, toothpaste, bottled water, sodas, juices, and many foods manufactured using artificially fluoridated water. With all these sources, you can easily exceed the recommended dose of daily fluoride consumption and start to see negative health effects. Even the American Dental Association recommends that infant formula be mixed with non-fluoridated water to make certain bottle-fed babies don't receive toxic levels of fluoride.[5]

Remember, fluoride is also added to most toothpaste, but with a bit of searching, you can find brands that have non-fluoride options, such as some varieties made by Tom's of Maine, USANA, and Coral LLC - Coral White Tea Tree Toothpaste.

Distilled water is a good choice for infants and children, or you can install a home filter system. Remember to consider filters for your showerheads as anything that goes on the skin can be found in the blood stream within twenty minutes. Here is the water filter that I use:

Pure Earth   www.pure-earth.com/fluoride-water-filters.htm

Digestion and Your Emotions

A little-known fact is that good digestion can make you happier, and not just because you're farting less! Your gut is sometimes referred to as the "second brain" because it produces about 85 percent of the serotonin used in the body. Remember, serotonin is that happiness hormone. Digestive issues relate to depression issues. So when you have cravings for carbs and sugar, it's your own body's way of trying to increase serotonin levels in the brain. By making your digestion more effective, you'll be helping your body have more stable levels of serotonin. If you are sensitive to sugar, you may have a lack of serotonin receptors in your brain. If you are faced with a plate of cookies or something sweet, can you eat one and walk away? If not, you may be sugar sensitive. Get the whole scoop on sugar sensitivity in my favorite sugar addict book, *Potatoes Not Prozac* by Caroline Des Maison.

I also offer a program that gets your gut healed and healthy in just four weeks. The program is found online and includes not only lots of useful information but also personal coaching with me. The best thing is, it's super simple to do. Here are the details:

Clear the Way to a Vibrant Life
30 day clean eating program

Recommended by Christiane Northup, M.D.

"It all starts with the gut! The 'Clear the Way' program is an effective and practical approach to gut health, without which, true health is not possible." —#1 *New York Times* Best Selling author Christiane

Northrup, M.D. *Author of Women's Bodies, Women's Wisdom, Mother Daughter Wisdom, The Wisdom of Menopause and Goddesses Never Age.*

Clear the Way Kit, includes
- Three Protein shake pouches (nine servings each)
- Twenty-eight day supply of Customized Nutritional Supplements
- Twenty-eight day supply of probiotic
- Twenty-eight day supply of digestive enzymes
- Fibergy (dietary fiber to add to your shakes)
- Program guide
- Three check-in calls with me
- Online membership program with videos, handouts and audios

This program guides you through a prep week and then four weeks of digestion and detox support. Here is a link with more program info: http://healthcoachdonna.com/clear-the-way

Action Items:

1. Drink more water.
2. Increase HCL in the stomach with digestive enzymes.
3. Add probiotics, prebiotics, and fiber to your daily routine.
4. Cut out toxic chemicals like soda and artificial sweeteners.
5. Get fluoride out of your daily routine.
6. Make a plan to repair your gut health.

Daily Intake Journal

What did you eat today?

Breakfast _____

_____

Lunch _____

_____

Dinner _____

Other _____

How are you feeling?

Did you experience any physical effects after a meal or snack?

How did you sleep last night?

What exercise did you do today?

Weekly Check-in

At the end of each week, take a moment to reflect and check in with your mind, body, and spirit. How are you feeling in each of these areas?

Rate any of the items listed below that you may be experiencing.

1=very slightly, 2=mild, 3=frequently, and 4=constantly

Add your ratings and make note of the total.

Head
- Headaches
- Dizziness
- Brain fog
- Puffy eyes

Nose
- Nasal congestion
- Excessive mucus
- Stuffy/runny nose
- Clear throat frequently

Lungs and skin

- Chest congestion
- Asthma or bronchitis
- Acne
- Hives, eczema, dry skin
- Excessive sweating

Emotions
- Food cravings
- Emotional eating
- Compulsive eating
- Mood swings
- Depression
- Anxiety
- Nervousness
- Irritability/short temper

Digestion
- Nausea/vomiting
- Diarrhea
- Constipation
- Bloating
- Belching/passing gas
- Heartburn/indigestion
- Intestinal/stomach pain
- Water retention/swelling

Energy
- Fatigue
- Lethargy
- Hyperactivity
- Restlessness
- Sleep quality

Muscles/joints
- ○ Pain/aching joints
- ○ Arthritis
- ○ Muscle stiffness
- ○ Muscle aches
- ○ Weak muscles

TOTAL:

****

[1] Jon Gabriel, *The Gabriel Method: The Revolutionary DIET-FREE Way to Totally Transform Your Body*, New York: Simon and Schuster, 2008), 119.

[2] Myron Wentz and David Wentz, *The Healthy Home: Simple Truths to Protect Your Family from Hidden Household Dangers* (New York: Vanguard Press, 2011).

[3] Ibid.

[4] Ibid.

[5] Ibid.

Week 5

Sleep and Stress

Stress! Who doesn't feel stressed these days? Stress affects how fat and sugar are processed in the body. It also affects weight gain, heart disease, hormones, and DNA. It depletes your body of magnesium, vitamin B, and vitamin C. It can shorten your life.

The crazy thing about stress is that it's perceived. By this I mean that you take in information and perceive the level of stress. A full email in-box can be stressful to some and no big deal to others. A single mom can juggle many things and feel in control while a stay-at-home mom with a nanny can feel overwhelmed. There is no judgment on who should feel more stressed, as stress is an individual issue.

If you weren't so stressed, you'd have time to relax and meditate! So what do you do about it? There are several things you can do to reduce your stress *response*. The first and most basic one I like is to stop and breathe. Yes, it's that simple.

When you are feeling stressed, stop and check your breathing. Is it shallow and only in the upper portion of your chest? Stop and notice it. Sometimes you may even catch yourself holding your breath. In that moment, stop whatever you are doing and take five deep belly breaths. Put one hand on your heart and the other on your belly and inhale while feeling your belly rise and fill with oxygen. Now release the breath fully and completely. Do this five times and you will start to connect the sympathetic nervous system (fight or flight) with the parasympathetic (calming) nervous system. Remember, we talked about that back in the digestion section. You can also have a little mantra going. As you inhale, say, "I feel calm," and with the exhale say, "I smile." Not only will you feel calm, but you'll actually start to smile, and that will set off another whole chemical reaction in the brain, which will leave you feeling happier. All that in only five breaths! Amazing.

Ever notice you tend to gain weight when you're stressed? Anxiety can cause late-night or mindless eating that adds pounds and inches to your body. If this sounds like you, keep reading, as I've got some great solutions for you to slow down, sleep better, and let go of those unwanted and unnecessary pounds. Here are five tips on how to reduce stress and anxiety-induced weight gain.

1. Don't eat when you're not hungry: First, figure out what your trigger is, what is causing you to eat continually throughout the day or late into the night. Before you reach for that next pretzel, ask yourself if you're hungry or if you're eating out of boredom. Maybe you feel you're lacking something and hoping food will fill the emptiness. The first step is to just identify the feeling that is triggering the eating. Then acknowledge the trigger. Next, keep a journal and write down your triggers. Identifying and acknowledging your triggers will help you to start shifting the behavior.

   Consuming sugar releases serotonin, the "feel good" hormone. So when you reach for the cookies, brownies, and such, you may be striving to feel happier in the moment. But if you are conscious of the connection between sweets, serotonin, and feeling better, you can help yourself feel better by naturally increasing your serotonin levels in healthier ways, such as going for a walk in nature and having a laugh with a friend.

2. Reduce your stress and anxiety: This can be done by engaging the sympathetic and parasympathetic nervous system as described earlier in this section.

If you enjoy regular meditation, yoga, exercise, dancing, or just walking in nature, you'll be pleased to know that all of these activities can reduce your stress response. Pick something you love and that brings you joy and figure out how to fit it into your daily life. That could mean just five minutes of meditation or working out per day. Don't make it a big deal, or you'll never get started.

3. Limit your alcohol: Save the alcohol until after you've eaten something with protein (e.g., nuts, turkey, cheese). All that sugar on an empty stomach will just spike your blood sugar levels. When your levels plummet, you'll end up ravenous! Alcohol also quells our inhibitions (it's harder to say "no" to yourself), and that often leads us to mindlessly snacking on chips and dip while we end up consuming larger quantities than planned. (Remember to drink water between alcoholic drinks as alcohol is dehydrating.) Try mixing a bit of seltzer with a small amount of fruit juice for a refreshing and satisfying drink. Staying hydrated will help you with any potential residual affects the next morning, and will also help you sleep better that night.

4. Eat regular, balanced meals: Start your day with breakfast within one hour of rising, and include protein in that and every meal throughout the day. If you need a snack, pair it with protein. So an apple goes with nuts, nut butter, or cheese. Eating within one hour of rising gets your blood sugar in a normal range and will help your energy throughout the day. Studies have shown that people who eat a protein breakfast eat 80 percent fewer calories throughout the day. Many of those extra calories are consumed between dinner and bedtime, so eat at least three, well-balanced meals through the day that include protein and lots of veggies. Keep refined carbohydrates to a minimum as they can trigger sugar cravings, which can be a very slippery slope.

5. Get enough sleep: Does the alarm go off and you're still sleepy? What is the right amount of sleep? It's more than most people get; seven to nine hours is ideal. Many people are running around sleep deprived and using massive amounts of caffeine

to make it through the day. Sleeping the *right* eight hours is also essential to balance. You have an internal clock that knows your ideal time sleep, eat, have sex, and have a bowel movement. Working in sync with your internal clock will help you feel well rested, digest your food better, and help your mood. Getting to bed between 9 and 10 p.m. is ideal. I know, you might think that sounds crazy, but my suggestion is to start getting ready for bed an hour before you actually want to sleep. Have a wind-down routine, lower the lights, and get off the electronics. If you are a night owl, then just start by going to bed fifteen minutes earlier per week. Make it a slow transition, and you will reap the benefits of a restful night's sleep. Caffeine can take about twelve hours to be processed through your body. So keep the coffee consumption to before 11 a.m. Get up between 5 and 6 a.m. Start your day with a cup of warm lemon water, and that will get your bowels moving. Then have breakfast between 7 and 9 a.m. and dinner before 7 p.m. By the way, the ideal time for sex is 7 to 9 p.m. I knew you were wondering that!

Sleep is another great way to lower your stress levels. The reason sleep is so key is that growth hormone is released while in deep REM sleep. This hormone helps reduce fat, increases your immune system function, and helps your liver function. Good liver function is key to keeping cholesterol levels in balance. Sleep deprivation increases the hunger hormone, which can cause you to overeat during the day. Lack of sleep decreases your vitamin D levels, which is linked to cancer, depression, and a host of other issues.

While you sleep, serotonin is released. That's the happiness hormone. Serotonin reduces cortisol levels, the stress hormone. Cortisol is released by the adrenal glands and assists you with energy. Too much cortisol throughout the day will increase your blood sugar levels and causes your body to store fat. It also decreases collagen, which will increase wrinkles in your face.

So, one of the best things you can do for stress is get more sleep (and meditate, as you learned in Week 1). If you don't sleep well, try melatonin supplements. My choice for sleep-aid supplementation is a multivitamin with antioxidants, clean fish oil, CoQ30, Hepasil DTX, and Proflavenal C (these are USANA brand). The last three are key for supporting your adrenals. When you've been under stress for an extended period of time, you are at risk of depleting your adrenal glands. These supplements will also support heart health, liver function, skin health, and immune function.

Don't let the search for perfection get in the way of achieving the good. The goal is progress, not perfection. Be patient with yourself and perhaps recruit an accountability partner who can support you while making lifestyle changes. Do something every day that makes you laugh or smile. Take a moment to be thankful and appreciative of all the abundance in your life. All these things "feed" you, and when you are nourished this way, food and drink fade in importance rather than being in the spotlight. When you are successful at putting your attention on the good things in life, you'll naturally start to notice more good stuff every day.

Stressful Thinking

We all have a running dialog in our brains. Changing that dialog will take some effort, but the benefits far outweigh the effort of input. Trust me, I've done this one. Our minds have about 60,000 thoughts per day. Of those thoughts, about 85 percent are negative and 90 percent are the same ones we had yesterday. The thing is, we have caveman DNA. That means that our brains filter for negative possibilities in order to survive. Now this made sense when we lived in caves and just stepping outside was a life-threatening challenge, but we don't live in that world anymore. Emails won't kill us. Another issue with negative thoughts is they lower your immune system. Researchers tested students in stressful test taking situations and found their immune systems to be lowered during the stressful period. [1]

Here's that fact again: changing your thoughts can also boost your immune system. That's why the nightly gratitude exercise is so important (see Week 1 in the meditation section). When you train your brain to look for positive experiences through the day, you will start to change the filter that your brain shifts information through. You want the positive filter to be more active than the negative filter. Yes, some people do have either a negative or positive view of life, but studies have shown that those views can be changed with daily effort.

Remember the exercise in Week 1 on self-limiting beliefs? Make sure you are doing something daily to change your thought patterns as they can also be physically damaging.

I'll let Jillian Michaels, personal trainer, tell you about the benefits of human growth hormone.

The hormone you always want more of

Growth hormone (sometimes referred to as HGH, for "human growth hormone") is something we all want more of. It builds muscle, burns fat, helps you resist heart disease, and protects your bones—among many other health benefits. By increasing your muscle mass, growth hormone raises your resting metabolic rate and gives you more power for your workouts. It also helps you tap into your fat stores for fuel and discourages your fat cells from absorbing or holding on to any fat floating around in your bloodstream.

In addition to these amazing feats, growth hormone helps your liver synthesize glucose, and it promotes gluconeogenesis, a really cool process that allows your body to create carbs out of protein. This helps you lose fat faster while providing your brain and other tissues with the energy they need.

As with so many other beneficial hormones, production of growth hormone declines with age, and many things we do speed the decline:

1. We deprive ourselves of good-quality sleep. Growth hormone is released in adults in an average of five pulses throughout the day, the largest of which happens during deep sleep. Shortchange yourself on sleep and you'll shortchange yourself on growth hormone.

2. We eat too many low-quality carbs. Refined carbs, such as those in white bread, white rice, and other processed foods, keep our blood sugar and insulin levels high, which suppresses the release of growth hormone. Protein, on the other hand, can facilitate the release of higher levels of growth hormone.

3. We don't exercise enough. When you don't exercise and your muscles become insulin-resistant, you increase your level of circulating insulin, which further suppresses growth hormone. You need to get off your butt and capitalize on this incredibly healthy hormone! One surefire way you can turn your body into a growth hormone factory is with intense exercise. During intense exercise, and especially during interval training, growth hormone encourages the body to use fat as its fuel instead of glucose. Not only does this help you burn fat while you exercise, but it stabilizes your blood glucose level so that you have the energy to *keep* exercising. [2]

Since I'm talking about fat here, I'd like to add a bit of information about cholesterol, as it's a very misunderstood fat. Here is a blog post I wrote in 2013. I hope it gives you a new perspective on cholesterol and statin drugs. If you have high cholesterol, the best thing to do is take a liver support supplement, such as USANA's Hepasil DTX. If you are currently on a statin, then you simply must take CoQ10 as the statins deplete it from your body and it is needed for a healthy brain.

The following is a newsletter I sent to my subscribers in 2013.
What you eat does not cause heart disease.
Are you serious?

I've just finished the most incredible book. So incredible, that I had to share my notes with all of you. Yes, it's longer than I normally write, but below are all the key points from Dr. Malcom Kendrick's *The Great Cholesterol Con*. If you have any interest in the details about the so-called science behind cholesterol and statin drugs, then I would highly recommend reading this book.

Here are the key points from the book:

After eleven years, the Surgeon General's office in the United States had found *no* evidence whatsoever to support the diet–heart hypothesis. If you want to read more on this, look at Gary Taubes "The Soft Science of Dietary Fat" published in *Science. That means, eat whole-fat, organic dairy, and eat the whole egg, yes the yellow part too.*

Long-term use of statins for primary prevention of heart disease produced a 1 percent greater risk of death over ten years versus placebo when the result of all the big controlled trials reported before 2000 were combined. Statins do not reduce mortality in men who do not *already* have diagnosed heart disease, which represents considerably more than 90 percent of the male population.

Statins not only have zero effect on overall mortality, they also have zero effect on reducing heart disease in women. So you get absolutely no benefits at all.

Statins do not reduce overall mortality in women.

Statins do not reduce overall mortality in men *without* heart disease.

Statins do not, therefore, reduce overall mortality in greater than 95 percent of the adult population.

Our brain needs fat to function. In fact, the brain contains over 25 percent of the total amount of cholesterol in the body and over 2 percent of the total weight of the brain is cholesterol. If you want the brain to function, this requires cholesterol. Without cholesterol, your brain cannot form synapses, and you can't think properly or remember anything.

In addition to cholesterol's critical function in synapse formation, it has now been found that a low cholesterol level leads to reduced serotonin levels in the brain. A low serotonin level is one of the key brain abnormalities involved in depression. This is why the most commonly used antidepressants are designed to boost serotonin levels.

Did you know that an early sign of cancer is low cholesterol levels? People with low cholesterol levels are at a much greater risk of dying of cancer. People with high cholesterol levels are less likely to die of cancer.

Some disturbing facts:

1. Statins cause cancer in animals.
2. There is some evidence that cancer deaths are increased in the statin trials, especially in those who are hyper-responders to statins.
3. A low cholesterol level is associated with a high risk of death from cancer.
4. It can take many, many years for cancer causing agents to reveal themselves.

CoQ10 is found in all cells everywhere in the body. It is found in particularly high concentrations in high-energy cells such as muscles, and especially in cardiac muscle cells where it plays a key role in the production of ATP. ATP is what fuels the cell. When ATP runs out, the cell dies. This is serious, especially in the heart muscle, the muscle that can never rest. Both human and animal studies have shown that reduced CoQ10 levels can lead to left and right-sided ventricular dysfunction (heart failure).

If low CoQ10 levels can lead to heart failure, and statins block the production of CoQ10, then statins could cause heart failure. Thus, adding CoQ10 to a statin makes perfect sense, does it not?

Statins reduce overall mortality in men with *existing* heart disease.

So what does cause heart disease?

1. Smoking. It increases cortisol levels and DHEA, the steroid hormone made in the adrenal glands in response to stress.

2. Lack of exercise. It's important to choose exercise that you enjoy. Human beings need some exercise; if they don't get it, they degenerate. They also become depressed, anxious, and unhappy.

3. Too much or too little alcohol. Small amounts of alcohol taken with friends or socially is healthy.

4. If you hate your job or have a bully for a boss. Don't be a victim or feel trapped. Assert yourself and ensure that people give you the respect that you deserve.

5. Lack of friendships. Make a new friend. Join a club. Find an area of life that you enjoy and can enjoy in the company of other people. Praise other people and try to compliment people more often. Look forward to something enjoyable every day, every month and every year.

There are differences between good stress and bad stress. I recommend watching "Stress: Portrait of a Killer" from National Geographic.

Sources of "good" stress:

Exercise
Massage
Singing
Rock climbing
Passing an exam
Clinching a successful business deal
Organizing a social event
Giving a well received lecture

Sources of "bad" stress:

Excessive, intense exercise in adverse conditions (e.g., working in a coal mine)
Cocaine use
Smoking
Major surgery/trauma
Steroid use
Bullying boss or colleague
Poor social network
Suffering racism

Money worries, long term debt

Okay, there you have it. If you're on a statin, you can stop without lowering the dosage first. If you don't eat fat, start. If you are on a statin and plan to continue taking it, then add a good nutritional supplement and CoQ10. I can help you with that, if you'd like.

Here is another resource with information about cholesterol and health:

www.westonaprice.org/know-your-fats/
importance-of-saturated-fats-for-biological-functions

If you want to know more about the potential damage caused by trans fats, just search for Mary Enig. You may never eat margarine again!

www.youtube.com/watch?v=5dpFFqN94JE

Dangers of Statin Drugs: What You Haven't Been Told About Popular Cholesterol-Lowering Medicines

www.westonaprice.org/cardiovascular-disease/
dangers-of-statin-drugs

Action Items:

1. Get aligned with your internal clock.
2. Get more sleep (seven to nine hours).
3. Figure out how to reduce your stress in the moment and in the long term.
4. If you're on a statin, take USANA's CoQ30.
5. Change negative thought patterns.

Daily Intake Journal

What did you eat today?

Breakfast _____

_____

Lunch _____

_____

Dinner _____

_____

Other _____

_____

How are you feeling?

Did you experience any physical effects after a meal or snack?

How did you sleep last night?

What exercise did you do today?

Weekly Check-in

At the end of each week, take a moment to reflect and check in with your mind, body, and spirit. How are you feeling in each of these areas?

Rate any of the items listed below that you may be experiencing.

1=very slightly, 2=mild, 3=frequently, and 4=constantly

Add your ratings and make note of the total.

Head
- Headaches
- Dizziness
- Brain fog
- Puffy eyes

Nose
- Nasal congestion
- Excessive mucus
- Stuffy/runny nose
- Clear throat frequently

Lungs and skin
- Chest congestion
- Asthma or bronchitis
- Acne
- Hives, eczema, dry skin
- Excessive sweating

Emotions
- Food cravings
- Emotional eating
- Compulsive eating
- Mood swings
- Depression
- Anxiety
- Nervousness
- Irritability/short temper

Digestion
- Nausea/vomiting
- Diarrhea
- Constipation
- Bloating
- Belching/passing gas
- Heartburn/indigestion
- Intestinal/stomach pain
- Water retention/swelling

Energy
- Fatigue
- Lethargy
- Hyperactivity
- Restlessness
- Sleep quality

Muscles/joints
- Pain/aching joints
- Arthritis
- Muscle stiffness
- Muscle aches
- Weak muscles

TOTAL:

****

[1] American Psychological Association, *Stress Weakens the Immune System* (February 2006), http://www.apa.org/research/action/immune.aspx.

[2] Jillian Michaels, *The Hormone You Always Want More Of*, http://www.jillianmichaels.com/fit/lose-weight/helpful-hormone.

WEEK 6

Exercise: Burn Fat, not Sugar

Burning fat is what you want. Fat is a better source of fuel than sugar. When your body burns sugar for fuel, it produces chemicals that cause inflammation and oxidative stress. When you burn fat, you have a body that you feel great in.

Nutrition, sleep, and reducing stress have all been covered in the previous weeks. Each of these areas will help your body become a fat burning machine. Now it's time to talk about exercise.

The easiest thing to start with is walking. Walking will help you burn fat, set your metabolism up for more effective fat burning, increase circulation, help with detoxification, stress reduction, and reduce the risk for cardiovascular disease, diabetes, cancer, and depression. It's a great place to begin if you don't already have a workout routine.

The keys to effective exercise are the following:

1. Do only twenty to thirty minutes a day. (Five to six days a week, at a consistent time.)
2. Make it fun and easy.
3. Make it fifteen seconds easier and you're more likely to do it. Saving fifteen seconds can look like putting on your workout clothes first thing in the morning.

One of the biggest mistakes people make is doing lots and lots of cardio to burn fat. Muscle mass decreases with age, approximately 6 to 10 percent per decade. So, by the age of forty, you've lost somewhere in the range of 40 percent of your muscle mass.

I've often heard from my patients "I haven't changed a thing and all of a sudden I have this mush around my middle." Well, the average weight gain per decade is about ten pounds. That's ten pounds of fat, not muscle. Think about a pound of butter and if you make it into a ball, it's about the size of a grapefruit. In comparison, one pound of muscle is about the size of a tangerine. The muscle is much denser and takes up less space in your body.

What happens to people is that they not only add fat per decade, but their muscle mass decreases with lack of exercise. This results in a body that is softer and mushier because the fat is taking up more space. This happens even if you don't gain weight, but with lack of exercise, your body stores fat.

Let's look at the numbers for metabolism and burning fat. Muscle can burn fifty calories per pound. What does this mean? Imagine two pounds of muscle (two tangerine-sized balls) and mush them out, one on each leg. At fifty calories burned per pound, that's a hundred extra calories burned each day!

At a hundred calories per day (remember, this is extra burning; you have added the muscle, now you just maintain it), how many calories is that in one month? A hundred calories a day for thirty days is an extra three thousand calories burned in just one month!

It takes 3,500 calories to burn up one pound of fat. If you added just two pounds of muscle, in one month you'd burn almost the equivalent of a pound of fat. That in itself should motivate you to get out there and build some muscle.

Strength training is done with some kind of resistance. That could be weights, your own body, or elastic bands. If you don't like the idea of lifting weights, there are plenty of possibilities that do not include lifting weights for strength training. Here is a link to fifty body weight exercise you can do anywhere: http://greatist.com/fitness/50-bodyweight-exercises-you-can-do-anywhere.

Building muscle is great. It increases your metabolism, burns more fat, makes you look more toned and leaner. Even if you just start with only ten minutes a day, that's an accomplishment.

Here is a quick, thirty-minute walking workout by fitness expert, Kathy Kaehler (http://www.kathykaehler.net/)

> 5 minutes: Walk at moderate pace, swing your arms to warm up.
>
> 1 minute: Do lunges or squats to warm up your lower body. Keep moving and don't hold the stretches as you want to warm up your body.
>
> 3 minutes: Power walk for 1 minute, taking exaggerated strides, longer than your normal stride. Keep a tall posture and look forward. Alternate between fast and normal pace.
>
> 5 minutes: Power surge for 1 minute of walking lunges. Lunge forward with your right leg, bending the knees at a 90 degree angle, then rise only slightly to bring your left leg forward into a lunge. Stay low to keep the tension on the thighs. Alternate between one minute of lunge walking and normal pace walking.
>
> 5 minutes: Return to the 1 minute of exaggerated strides and 1 minute of normal pace walking.
>
> 4 minutes: Repeat walking lunges and normal pace walking for 1 minute each.
>
> 5 minutes: Repeat exaggerated strides and normal pace walking.
>
> 2 minutes: End with a cool down stride and easy stretching.

This workout will get you moving, burning calories, and firming your lower body. Once you get comfortable with these moves, I would suggest adding light hand weights and doing combination moves such as bicep curls while lunging, or overhead presses while walking. The possibilities are endless. Just remember to have fun with it.

Here are a few options from fitness trainer and expert, Dot Spaet:

www.fitnessbydot.com/homepage.htm

www.youtube.com/watch?v=x82oRLvgSr8

This is five-minute office fitness. www.youtube.com/watch?v=1TltoZ2vDO8

A yoga routine that is somewhat challenging, four minutes, and a great workout!

fitnessbydot.com/abwork.htm

This is six-ab moves, takes about twelve minutes to watch and learn them, and it only takes about six minutes to do all of them.

Action Items:

1. Move your body. Start with five to ten minutes per day and slowly work up to twenty to thirty minutes, five to six times per week.
2. Continue to drink plenty of water.
3. Continue with your food log and meal planning.
4. Continue to get seven to nine hours of sleep per night.

Daily Intake Journal

What did you eat today?

Breakfast _____

_____

Lunch _____

_____

Dinner _____

_____

Other _____

_____

How are you feeling?

Did you experience any physical effects after a meal or snack?

How did you sleep last night?

What exercise did you do today?

Weekly Check-in

At the end of each week, take a moment to reflect and check in with your mind, body, and spirit. How are you feeling in each of these areas?

Rate any of the items listed below that you may be experiencing.

1=very slightly, 2=mild, 3=frequently, and 4=constantly

Add your ratings and make note of the total.

Head
- o Headaches
- o Dizziness
- o Brain fog
- o Puffy eyes

Nose
- o Nasal congestion
- o Excessive mucus
- o Stuffy/runny nose
- o Clear throat frequently

Lungs and skin
- o Chest congestion
- o Asthma or bronchitis
- o Acne
- o Hives, eczema, dry skin
- o Excessive sweating

Emotions
- o Food cravings
- o Emotional eating
- o Compulsive eating
- o Mood swings
- o Depression
- o Anxiety
- o Nervousness
- o Irritability/short temper

Digestion
- o Nausea/vomiting
- o Diarrhea
- o Constipation
- o Bloating
- o Belching/passing gas
- o Heartburn/indigestion
- o Intestinal/stomach pain
- o Water retention/swelling

Energy
- ○ Fatigue
- ○ Lethargy
- ○ Hyperactivity
- ○ Restlessness
- ○ Sleep quality

Muscles/joints
- ○ Pain/aching joints
- ○ Arthritis
- ○ Muscle stiffness
- ○ Muscle aches
- ○ Weak muscles

TOTAL:

Week 7

Happiness

Happiness is something I often talk about with my patients. I like to remind them, and you, that whatever you focus on expands. Complaining only attracts more opportunities to complain. Appreciation brings more good stuff to appreciate.

Take a moment to write down three things you appreciate in your life right now.

Remember the ship heading for Europe and the fact that if it made a one-degree course change, it could end up in Africa? I want to remind you that you can make a small shift that creates huge changes in your life. What are some small changes you can implement in your life right now that will give you big results in just a few short months? Some of those changes are actually all the things you've been doing over the last six weeks of this program: sleep, exercise, gratitude, and meditation. These are all small changes that, over time, will yield large rewards.

When I coach people through my five-day carb cleanse, I talk to them about Day 3 and the challenges that might come up. By Day 3, serotonin is coming into balance and they often feel a bit depressed or angry as a result. Remember, carbs and sugars boost serotonin in the short term. I talk to them about what they can do to naturally boost their serotonin levels.

Natural Ways To Boost Serotonin Levels

1. A food plan in place, so healthy food is on hand
2. Daily exercise
3. Mindfulness—meditation or praying or nature
4. Full-spectrum light in your home and office
5. Body work (massage)
6. Friendships
7. Sleep (seven to nine hours)
8. Quick bursts of positive emotion, YouTube (check out Jessica's daily affirmations https://www.youtube.com/watch?v=qR3rK0kZFkg), or photos that bring joy
9. Daily vitamin supplements
10. Five minutes of daily meditation focused on breath
11. Anticipation of fun activities (plan something fun weekly)

Dan Buettner has spent years studying what makes people happy. He has developed a quiz, the True Happiness Compass, at www.bluezones.com, that you can take for free online. It takes about five minutes and the questions are surprising. When you're done, you'll get personalized recommendations for boosting your happiness. Have fun with it!

The Value Of Positive Emotions

In her article, "The Value of Positive Emotions," Barbara L. Fredrickson describes the following study showing the impact positive emotions can have on our lives. Back in the 1930s, some young Catholic nuns were asked to write short personal essays about their lives. They described edifying events in their childhood, the schools they attended, their religious experiences, and the influences that led them to the convent. Although the essays may have been initially used to assess each nun's career path, the documents were eventually archived and largely forgotten. More than sixty years later, the nuns' writings surfaced again when three psychologists at the University of Kentucky reviewed the essays as part of a larger study on aging and Alzheimer's disease. Deborah Danner, David Snowdon, and Wallace Friesen read the nun's biographical sketches and scored them for positive emotional content, recording instances of happiness, interest, love, and hope. What they found was remarkable: The nuns who expressed the most positive emotions lived up to ten years longer than those who expressed the fewest. This gain in life expectancy is considerably larger than the gain achieved by those who quit smoking. [1]

All of this suggests that we need to develop methods to experience more positive emotions more often and appears to answer the question, "What good is it to think about the good in the world?" Positive meaning can be obtained by finding benefits within adversity, by infusing ordinary events with meaning and by effective problem solving. You can find benefits in a grim world, for instance, by focusing on the new-found strengths and resolve you have discovered within yourself and others. You can infuse ordinary events with meaning by expressing appreciation, love, and gratitude, even for simple things. And you can find positive meaning through problem solving by supporting compassionate acts toward people in need. Although the active ingredient within growth and resilience may be positive emotions, the leverage point for accessing these benefits is finding positive meaning.

The mind can be a powerful ally. As John Milton told us, "The mind is its own place, and in itself can make a heaven of hell, a hell of heaven."

Shawn Achor's Six Exercises For Happiness

Shawn Achor, author of *The Happiness Advantage*, says you can rewire your brain to make yourself happy by practicing simple happiness exercises. Within thirty days, those habits change the neuropathways of our brains and turn us into lifelong optimists.

These six daily happiness exercises are proven to make anyone, from a four-year old to an eighty-four-year old, happy, or simply happier, Achor says,

1. Gratitude exercises. Write down three things you're grateful for that occurred over the last twenty-four hours. They don't

have to be profound. It could be a really good cup of coffee or the warmth of a sunny day.

2. The doubler. Take one positive experience from the past twenty-four hours and spend two minutes writing down every detail about that experience. As you remember it, your brain labels it as meaningful and deepens the imprint.

3. The fun fifteen. Do fifteen minutes of a fun cardio activity, like gardening or walking the dog, every day. The effects of daily cardio can be as effective as taking an antidepressant.

4. Meditation. Every day take two minutes to stop whatever you're doing and concentrate on breathing. Even a short mindful break can result in a calmer, happier you.

5. Conscious act of kindness. At the start of every day, send a short email or text praising someone you know. Our brains become addicted to feeling good by making others feel good.

6. Deepen social connections. Spend time with family and friends. Our social connections are one of the best predictors for success and health, and even life expectancy. [2]

Read the full article here: http://www.cbc.ca/player/News/ID/2665132971/

Action Items:

1. Daily gratitude: write down three things every twenty-four hours.

2. Continue with daily meditation, breathing, and do fifteen minutes of cardio per day.

3. Find one thing to do daily to boost your serotonin naturally.

Daily Intake Journal

What did you eat today?

Breakfast _____

_____

Lunch _____

_____

Dinner _____

_____

Other _____

_____

How are you feeling?

Did you experience any physical effects after a meal or snack?

How did you sleep last night?

What exercise did you do today?

Weekly Check-in

At the end of each week, take a moment to reflect and check in with your mind, body, and spirit. How are you feeling in each of these areas?

Rate any of the items listed below that you may be experiencing.

1=very slightly, 2=mild, 3=frequently, and 4=constantly

Add your ratings and make note of the total.

Head
- Headaches
- Dizziness
- Brain fog
- Puffy eyes

Nose
- Nasal congestion
- Excessive mucus
- Stuffy/runny nose
- Clear throat frequently

Lungs and skin
- Chest congestion
- Asthma or bronchitis
- Acne
- Hives, eczema, dry skin
- Excessive sweating

Emotions
- Food cravings
- Emotional eating
- Compulsive eating
- Mood swings
- Depression
- Anxiety
- Nervousness
- Irritability/short temper

Digestion
- Nausea/vomiting
- Diarrhea
- Constipation
- Bloating
- Belching/passing gas
- Heartburn/indigestion
- Intestinal/stomach pain
- Water retention/swelling

Energy
- o Fatigue
- o Lethargy
- o Hyperactivity
- o Restlessness
- o Sleep quality

Muscles/joints
- o Pain/aching joints
- o Arthritis
- o Muscle stiffness
- o Muscle aches
- o Weak muscles

TOTAL:

****

[1] Barbara L. Fredrickson, "The Value of Positive Emotions," *American Scientist* (July-August 2003): 330–335.

[2] Joanna Roumeliotis, Joanna. "Happiness Is a Choice Not a Pursuit, Psychologist Advises" *CBC News* (April 2015), http://www.cbc.ca/news/health/shawn-achor-s-6-exercises-for-happiness-1.3040937.

WEEK 8

Put it all together

Over the past seven weeks, you have made many small and some big changes in your life. I suggest you take a moment to have gratitude and appreciation for your self and the work you've done. Making lifestyle changes takes commitment and focus. I congratulate you for completing the program and encourage you to stay on course. Over time, these changes you've made will just be habits and part of who you are. Below is a daily outline that will help you structure your day and easily implement the changes you've made over the last seven weeks. Congratulations and keep going!

5–7 am
Rise and shine.
Start with two to ten minutes of meditation.
Drink a cup of warm lemon water before anything else.
Eat breakfast with protein or drink a USANA protein shake.
Take your AM nutritional supplements.
Engage in ten to twenty minutes of exercise of your choice.
Drink a glass of water.

12–1 pm
Lunch with lots of veggies and some protein or a shake.
Drink a glass of water after eating.

2 pm
Drink a glass of water.

3 pm
If you need a snack, make sure it includes protein.
Drink a glass of water.

5–7 pm
Eat dinner.
Remember to have half to two-thirds your plate in veggies and include
a lean protein.
Drink a glass of water after eating.
Take your evening supplements.

9 pm
Turn off all electronics by 9 p.m. and start a bedtime routine such as
gentle stretching, Chi machine, hot tea, and an old fashioned book (not
an electronic reader).
A warm bath with Epsom salts is a great way to relax and detoxify
your body.

10 pm
Practice meditation and gratitude.
Take your liver-support supplement and turn the lights out.

Do this routine with no sugar and no carbs for at least ten days. Once
you've completed the ten days, on the eleventh day, you can have a
meal with some carbohydrates such as rice or pasta. This will actually
help reset your metabolism and reignite your fat-burning hormones.
It triggers a very short, lasting spike in insulin, which is the signal
your body waits for to ramp up your metabolism. After the first ten
days, you can have a carb portion (a third of a cup of brown rice, for
example) to your meal every fourth day. To be clear, a carb portion is
not an entire plate of pasta.

Along with the meditation, breathing, and exercise to help with stress,
I strongly suggest doing something fun at least three times a week.
This can be anything that brings you joy and helps you relax. Fun is

any activity that makes you lose track of time while you're doing it and you don't want it to end.

My intention with this guide is to make it simple and easy to implement lifestyle changes. I hope that is what your experience has been. If you have any need for additional support or have questions, feel free to contact me at Donna@DonnaAcupuncture.com. Here's to a happier, healthier, and more vibrant life.

Resources

Some of the foods include meat. If you are a vegetarian, just substitute with tofu, beans, or tempeh as you desire. The midmorning snack is optional or can be eaten later in the day, but not too late to push your dinner later than 7 p.m. Use the template below to give you an idea of how to plan your meals. Do this weekly and prep as much in advance as possible. The suggested meals will give you a general idea of how to prepare the dish. You can also look up new recipes online or use your favorite recipes.

Day 1	Day 2	Day 3	Day 4	Day 5	Day 6	Day 7
Veggie omelet 1 piece of fruit in season	Chia pudding	Shake	Two fried eggs with leftover veggies and turkey bacon	Shake	Scrambled eggs with cottage cheese	Tofu scramble
Snack	Snack	Snack	Snack	Snack	Snack	Snack
Salad/ veggies/ beans	Dinner leftovers with salad	Tuna salad with celery and tomatoes	Turkey burger and salad	Salad with veggies	Leftover soup	Leftover green beans and salad
Chicken with steamed seasonal veggies or beans *Prep chia pudding	Grilled or baked fish with veggies	Chickpea salad/ steamed broccoli Protein of your choice	Veggie stir-fry *Prep extra veggies for lunch	Spinach and lentil soup	Grilled fish Steamed green beans	Veggie soup

Breakfast suggestions

- USANA shake mix blended with frozen banana and walnuts
- USANA shake blended with frozen berries
- Frittata. Whisk three eggs with whole milk, toss in veggies of your choice and seasonings. Pour into greased glass pie pan. Bake for about 30 minutes at 350 degrees Fahrenheit.
- Huevos rancheros. Sauté black beans with onions and cumin. Fry eggs. Serve beans, egg, and full-fat, organic cheese on top of warm organic corn tortilla. Serve with fresh salsa if desired or just chopped tomatoes, onions, cilantro, and jalapenos.
- Fried eggs with sautéed greens (e.g., kale, chard, arugula) and turkey bacon.
- Egg and tofu scramble. Scramble two eggs with one package of drained and crumbled tofu, chopped red pepper, mushrooms, and turmeric. Serve with salsa.

- Two poached eggs served on zucchini and topped with salsa with half a grapefruit or melon of your choice.
- Eggs Florentine (one or two poached eggs served on half a cup of spinach sautéed in olive oil.
- Chia pudding. In a mason jar or something with a lid, add one cup of milk of your choice, whisk one tablespoon of almond butter, four tablespoons of chia seeds, one teaspoon of honey or maple syrup, then top with frozen raspberries and walnuts. Close tightly and shake well. Put in fridge overnight and enjoy from the jar in the morning.
- USANA shake blended with two tablespoons of tahini (sesame seed butter), half a banana, one small apple, two tablespoons of chia seeds, and cinnamon.

Snack suggestions

- Cheese (organic, full fat) with a handful of raw almonds
- Veggies of your choice with almonds or nuts of your choice
- Whole apple with a handful of raw nuts
- One cup of organic, full-fat Greek yogurt
- Any fruit with a protein (nuts or cheese)
- Hardboiled egg
- Apple with nut butter
- Carrots and one tablespoon of hummus
- Roasted chickpeas
- Kale chips

Salad suggestions

Green salad
Leaf lettuce, raw mushrooms, tomato, avocado, scallions, chickpeas, turkey, or chicken

Combine salad ingredients and olive oil and lemon juice

Chef's salad
Meat of your choice, hardboiled egg, mixed veggies, cottage cheese.
Toss with olive oil and lemon juice.

Tomato salad
Chop or slice a variety of seasonal tomatoes and toss with olive oil
and seasoning.

Tuna salad
Albacore tuna packed in water or leftover fresh tuna steak, chopped
celery, and mayo.

Chickpea salad
Mix drained garbanzo beans, kidney beans, chopped celery, olive oil,
and fresh chopped bell pepper.

Cabbage salad
Grate green and red cabbage. Toss with fennel, salt, and olive oil.

Spinach salad
Toss fresh spinach with mushrooms, red onion, hardboiled eggs,
chicken or cottage cheese, and red wine vinegar/olive oil.

Beet salad
Slice cooked beets and toss with onion, olive oil, salt, and apple cider
vinegar.

Antipasto salad
Arrange sliced ham, red peppers, tomatoes, Kalamata olives,
cucumbers, two slices of mozzarella cheese, lettuce, and garbanzo
beans on a plate and drizzle with olive oil.

Chicken or tofu salad
Mix with mayo, mustard, curry celery, and currants.

Cucumber salad
Dice cucumber, onion, celery, avocado, and toss with chopped cashews, cilantro, greens of your choice (kale, spinach, lettuce), and lemon juice/olive oil.

Dinner suggestions

- Chicken or beans served with your choice of steamed vegetable
- Grilled chicken served with salsa (chopped onions, tomatoes, jalapeno pepper, cilantro, and lime)
- Black beans seasoned with cumin, cilantro and onions
- Baked halibut with capers, olives, olive oil, and lemon juice. Bake 30 minutes at 400 degrees Fahrenheit.
- Turkey burger
- Grilled tempeh
- Grilled or baked salmon
- Black or pinto beans, grilled vegetables, tomato salsa, and guacamole served on lettuce.
- Sauté veggies and meat of your choice and serve wrapped in brown rice tortilla.

Veggie suggestions

- Seasonal veggies can be steamed, tossed in a skillet with olive oil, or tossed with olive oil and baked 20 minutes at 375 degrees Fahrenheit.
- Baked sweet potato.
- Stir-fry broccoli, snow peas, scallions, and carrots in sesame oil and tamari.
- Sauté fresh green beans with onion and garlic.
- Steam Brussels sprouts and toss with pine nuts and olive oil.
- Steam cauliflower and then mash like potatoes. Season and serve.
- Cube various seasonal veggies, toss with olive oil and tamari, place on skewers, and grill.

- Roast root veggies with olive oil, garlic, and rosemary, 20-40 minutes at 400 degrees Fahrenheit.
- Cauliflower rice. Place cauliflower in food processor and pulse until grainy like rice. Sauté onions in olive oil. Add cauliflower and cook until tender. Salt and pepper to taste.
- Sweet potato fries. Peel and thinly slice sweet potatoes. Toss with olive oil, sea salt, and rosemary. Place on baking sheet in oven for about 20 minutes at 400 degrees Fahrenheit.

Soup suggestions

- **Swiss Chard and White Bean Soup**

  1 bunch Swiss chard
  1 small onion, chopped
  3 cloves minced garlic
  4 cups vegetable or low sodium chicken stock
  2 cups cooked white beans (can be canned or fresh)

  Sauté onion and garlic in olive oil; add four cups of stock and bring to boil; add one bunch of chopped Swiss chard, reduce heat, cover and simmer chard until soft (ten minutes); add cooked white beans.

- **Lentil/Spinach Soup**

  1 small package dry lentils
  1 small onion, chopped
  1 stalk celery, chopped
  1 carrot, sliced
  1 cup chopped tomatoes
  4 cups vegetable broth
  1 bunch fresh spinach, stemmed and chopped

  Sauté onion, garlic, celery in olive oil. Add chopped carrot, chopped tomatoes, and simmer five minutes. Add lentils and vegetable broth; cover and simmer about thirty minutes or until lentils are soft. Add the chopped spinach and simmer five minutes. Serve with parmesan cheese, if desired.

- **Basic Veggie Soup**

  1/4 lb turkey bacon; if desired, can use tofu or tempeh
  2 medium onions, chopped
  1 clove garlic, minced
  1/2 cup chopped celery
  1 sliced carrot
  1 cup chopped cabbage
  1 cup spinach, stemmed and chopped
  1/2 cup peas
  1/4 cup chopped fresh parsley
  6 cups veggie or chicken broth
  1/2 teaspoon thyme
  1/2 teaspoon basil
  1 cup cooked white beans, can use canned
  Parmesan or pesto

  Sauté vegetables with tofu or bacon until tender. Add the broth and spices and simmer for forty minutes. Add the cooked beans can cook five to ten minutes more. Serve with parmesan or fresh pesto, if desired.

Chia Breakfast Pudding

  1 cup almond milk (or other milk of choice)
  1 tablespoon almond butter (or nut butter of choice)
  4 tablespoon chia seeds
  1–2 teaspoon honey or maple syrup, optional
  Handful of fresh or frozen raspberries or other berry
  Handful of walnuts or other nut

  In a container or pint Mason jar, whisk together milk and nut butter. Add chia and stir to combine well. Add fruit on top. Shake the jar to make sure all the ingredients are dispersed throughout the liquid. Cover and place in fridge overnight.

What Are Your Kids Eating for Breakfast?
This is a blog I posted on February 14, 2011.

I volunteer in my son's first and second grade class. The other morning, I was noticing that several kids were just unable to focus. Earlier in the morning I had seen one child eating a chocolate croissant at his desk. When asked, he stated that it was his breakfast. So I got the idea to ask all the children who couldn't focus, what they ate for breakfast.

Here is what I got:

1. Waffles with jam
2. Nothing
3. Cereal

Each of these meals is highly glycemic. That means that their blood sugar was boosted, then dropped to a lower level than before eating. That leaves their brain foggy and unable to function. The truth is, many people don't understand the glycemic index of foods or how carbs and fruit is like eating a bowl of sugar.

One parent I spoke to explained that cereal is easy; they can do it themselves. She was open to ideas, but they had to be quick in order for her to consider it doable.

Why? Why have our meals gotten to quick things eaten while running out the door? Is fifteen minutes too much to spend preparing a hot, well-balanced breakfast? What if you spent some time on the weekends teaching your child to cook simple meals? I'm just not sure why mealtime has dropped to a lower priority than almost anything else in our lives.

So, here are some quick, simple, low-glycemic breakfast ideas.

Cottage cheese, almonds and fresh fruit.

Scrambled eggs with sprouted grain toast

Quinoa Porridge
Make quinoa with milk instead of water as directed; we like almond milk. This can be made several days in advance and then just reheated on the stove top in the morning by adding a little more milk. My son enjoys this just like oatmeal and served with whole fat, organic Greek yogurt, a drizzle of honey or real maple syrup, and some almonds.

French Toast
This is a great treat to eat during the week. Use sprouted bread, like Ezekiel 4:9 or Trader Joe's Daily Bread. You can mix the egg with some almond milk and serve with organic Greek yogurt or cheese, a drizzle of honey or real maple syrup, and some almonds. To make this really quick and easy, make it on a weekend and make extra, freezing the leftovers. Just heat up a slice from the freezer, and you've got a speedy breakfast. Even kids can do it by themselves!

Toad in a Hole
Take a piece of sprouted-grain or gluten-free bread and cut out a small circle in the middle. Put some butter in a frying pan and melt. Place the bread in the pan and cook, just slightly. Put a little more butter in the pan and cook the other side of the bread. Take out the circle of bread, crack an egg, and drop it in the hole to cook. Once the egg is set, use a spatula to flip the egg and cook completely. Serve with the circle of bread on top.

Be creative and have fun. Eat your breakfast and feel energized throughout the morning. Remember, mom always said that breakfast is the most important meal of the day. Boy, was she right!

I Love (Gluten-Free) Waffles ...

But, I don't like the spike in blood sugar and the cravings I get after eating them. Even the gluten-free flour waffles I've made in the past left me feeling a bit woosey within an hour of eating them.

So, I was craving a good waffle and decided I needed to develop a better one. I used a few of my gluten-free recipe books and my paleo cookbook to come up with one that I absolutely loved. I felt full after eating them, and I had sustained energy with no lingering cravings.

My recipe uses buckwheat flour rather and wheat flour. Buckwheat has compounds such as rutin, which are helpful in maintaining an even blood glucose level after eating.

I grew up eating waffles with cheese melted in them. Yes, that sounds weird to most, but it gives the best flavor, as you have the combination of sweet and savory. I think it comes from our Dutch ancestors as they combine pancakes with cheese and meat. My father said his father made them that way, and he has no idea where he learned it from. So enjoy my family tradition and add some cheese to your waffles (or pancakes).

I like a good, sharp cheddar. I also like it because it adds a bit more protein to the meal and helps with insulin response and blood-sugar levels.

Once the waffles are finished cooking, open the iron and place a few slices of your favorite cheese on one half. Then take the other half and fold it over the cheese. Then close the waffle iron and let it sit for a minute or two while the cheese melts. Trust me, you'll love them this way.

Carbs for breakfast can speed up your metabolism if they are eaten with the right combo of protein.

If you're a fan of waffles or pancakes, give this a try, and I would love to know what you think of it. Bon appetit!

Gluten-Free Buckwheat Waffles

Dry ingredients:

1 1/2 cups buckwheat flour
1/3 cup coconut flour
1/4 cup almond meal
1 1/2 teaspoon baking powder
1/2 teaspoon baking soda
1/2 teaspoon sea salt
Dash cinnamon
Dash nutmeg

Wet ingredients:

2 tablespoon ground chia seeds
1/4 cup hot water
1 mashed banana
1 1/2 cups almond milk
2 tablespoon melted coconut oil
1 tablespoon maple syrup (the real stuff)
1 egg
Heat the waffle iron and spray with coconut oil.

Whisk together all the dry ingredients. In a separate bowl, whisk the egg and add all the ingredients except the water and chia seeds. In a small bowl, whisk the hot water and chia seeds, then add to the wet ingredients. Whisk the wet ingredients until everything is thoroughly incorporated. Add the wet ingredients to the dry and use a hand mixer to blend. If the batter is too thick, add a bit more milk until you've got a good consistency.

Add the batter to the hot waffle iron, gently spreading the mixture around the whole surface. These waffles don't spread like regular batter, so you'll need to do it in advance. Also, these will take longer to cook, more like ten minutes rather than five. Be patient and let them cook through. Freeze the extras and use them for a quick week day breakfast.

Makes about four waffles. Enjoy!

Kasha Cereal

It may sound like a grain, but it's actually a fruit seed of the buckwheat plant. It's related to rhubarb and sorrel, making it a great substitute for grains, especially for those avoiding gluten. The soft white seed has a mild flavor, but when toasted, the flavor becomes much more distinct and intense. I make a batch of this each week and keep in the fridge for a quick and easy breakfast served with almond milk or yogurt or eaten dry as a snack.

Ingredients

- 4 cups raw buckwheat groats
- 3/4 cup raw almond butter
- 3/4 cup chopped raw walnuts
- 3/4 cup raw pumpkin seeds (pepitas)
- 3 tablespoons real maple syrup
- 1 teaspoon cinnamon
- 1 teaspoon sea salt
- 3/4 cup dried currants
- ¾ cup unsweetened, shredded coconut

Preheat oven to 300°F. Spread raw buckwheat groats across a large cookie sheet and bake for about forty minutes, shuffling them around about halfway through, until slightly golden. While the groats are cooking, mix all other ingredients in a large glass bowl. When the groats are done, immediately mix them in the bowl with the other ingredients. It may take a bit of effort to get the groats thoroughly coated. Let cool to room temperature Place in a glass jar or large glass container and store in the fridge. You can use any nuts, dried fruit, and nut butter that you prefer. Start with my version and then make variations according to your taste.

Updated Granola Recipe

3 cups gluten-free rolled oats
2 cups raw nuts of your choice
1 cup sliced almonds
1 cup coconut flakes
1/2 cup ground flax or chia seeds
1/2 cup almond meal
1/4 cup brown sugar
1 teaspoon sea salt
1/3 cup coconut oil and butter, melt a little of both to make 1/3 cup
1/4 cup maple syrup

Mix all the dry ingredients and then add the wet. Toss until everything is coated with the oil and syrup. Spread out on a cookie sheet. I use two. Cook for one hour and fifteen minutes at 250°F. Stir every fifteen minutes. Cool and enjoy.

Fish Tacos

Coating

1/2 almond meal
3/4 cup unsweetened shredded coconut
1/4 teaspoon freshly ground black pepper
1/2 teaspoon turmeric
1/2 teaspoon paprika
1/4 teaspoon sea salt
Fish
1–2 lbs. firm white fish or chicken cut into small strips (I like Dover sole)
sesame oil for pan

Place almond meal and remaining coating ingredients in a shallow dish and mix to combine. Rinse the fish with cold water and leave damp but not soaked. Toss each fish strip in coating. Heat the oil in skillet. Just use enough to coat the bottom of a cast iron skillet. You'll need to add more if you are doing more than one batch of fish. Also, you might need to add a bit extra when you turn the fish to cook on the second side. You don't want to deep fry it, just enough oil to cook it evenly. Brown the fish and flip, about four minutes per side. Turn fish only once.

Place the cooked fish in warm corn tortillas. It should make about eight to ten small tortillas. Serve with salsa, salad, avocado, or any other favorite taco toppings. Enjoy!

Sauerkraut Benefits and How to Make It

I love sauerkraut. I especially enjoy it when it's spicy. Sauerkraut is fermented cabbage and really great for gut health. Fermenting your foods changes the chemistry of them. As a result, beneficial bacteria is produced. That bacteria can improve your digestion, your immune system, and endocrine function. Fermentation has been used for years to preserve veggies and other perishable foods for long periods. Your immune health is ruled by your gut health. When you eat fermented foods, the bacteria take up residence in your gut lining. They act like the first line of defense with bad bacteria or toxins. Cabbage is also high in vitamin A, C, iron, and fiber. Other than my twelve-year-old, who can't stand the smell, it's really a great thing for overall health. I suggest eating a couple of tablespoons with each meal.

Sauerkraut has become enormously popular in health food stores. But you do not have to pay those high prices for basically shredded cabbage and salt.

How to make sauerkraut

Shred 1 head of cabbage
Massage with 1 tablespoon of sea salt
Add 1–2 tablespoons of fennel
Add 1 fresh, chopped jalapeno pepper (optional spice)
Put into jar and press down until you see the juices coming up

Cover with cabbage leaves. Leave on the counter for three to seven days depending on how fermented you like the flavor. Once it's how you like it, remove the top cabbage leaves and any top layer that molded. Please in fridge and enjoy.

Watch my video for a demo on how easy it really is: https://youtu.be/ggQxb5CkbvM

Chia Chocolate Pudding

- 1 1/2 cups almond milk
- 1/3 cup chia seeds
- 1/4 cup unsweetened cocoa powder
- 3 tablespoons of maple syrup or 6 pitted dates
- 1/2 teaspoon ground cinnamon
- 1/4 teaspoon sea salt

Add all ingredients, in the order listed, in a blender. Blend until completely smooth and creamy. Pour into single serving bowls or jars, cover, and put in the fridge over night. Serve with fresh berries, if they are in season, or sweetened coconut flakes if desired.

Thanksgiving Cranberry Sauce

I love cranberry sauce, but not the jelly my mom used to serve from a can that came out in the tube shape with the can rings. You know what I'm talking about. Well, here is my cranberry relish recipe that I make every year for Thanksgiving. It's really more like a chutney, as it's a bit tart. I suggest you make it a day in advance as it sets up nicely over night in the fridge. Enjoy.

Cranberry Chutney

1 cup sugar; this can be raw or mixed with honey or maple syrup
1/2 cup dry red wine
2 bags organic cranberries
1/4 cup apple cider vinegar
1 granny smith apple
2 tablespoons freshly grated ginger
juice and grated zest of 1 orange
1/3 cup dried currants
1 to 2 tablespoons of cornstarch or arrowroot mixed in 1/4 cup water

In a medium saucepan combine sugar and wine. Bring to boil and reduce heat to medium and simmer, covered for five minutes. Add all the remaining ingredients except the currants. Cook until cranberries have popped, about ten minutes. Remove from heat. Stir in arrowroot/water and currants. Let cool and then place in glass container and refrigerate overnight.

It's an Antioxidant and Anti-inflammatory: Golden Milk

This recipe is from Sanoviv Medical Institute. I know you'll love it. Golden milk is an Ayurvedic healing tea where the main ingredient is turmeric. You may know turmeric from such foods as curries. It's has many healing properties with its active ingredient curcumin. It's an antioxidant and anti-inflammatory. It has been shown to help cancers, heart disease, type 2 diabetes, Crohn's disease, psoriasis, atopic dermatitis, and arthritis. You only need to drink a small amount. We were served this daily around 10 a.m., and it was such a treat. Hope you enjoy it.

1/4 cup water
1/8 teaspoon turmeric
1 cup almond or other nut milk
1–2 tablespoons almond oil (optional)
Pinch of cardamom and cinnamon
Raw honey to taste

Boil water and turmeric over medium heat for eight minutes. In another pan, boil nut milk and remove from heat. Add almond oil, cardamom, and honey. Combine with the water. Optionally, you can put it in a blender and blend until frothy and serve with a pinch of cinnamon. Enjoy!

Resources I love

Daily OM.com
Happify.com
The Happiness Advantage by Shawn Achor
Brené Brown's Whole Hearted Living
I keep a running list updated on my website at:
http://healthcoachdonna.com/free-resources-2

All About GLUTEN
from Sanoviv Medical Institute

What is Gluten?

Gluten is the major protein component of certain grains such as wheat, rye and barley. Most experts agree that this is a very difficult protein for human digestive tracts to break down. As such, it can be the root cause of a number of health problems in the body. The following is a list of symptoms for which gluten may be the culprit:

Digestive: bloating and/or gas, constipation and/or diarrhea, nausea, weight problems, iron-deficiency anemia, leaky gut (also known as intestinal permeability)
Neurological: headaches/migraines, memory problems, joint pains or aches, fibromyalgia, brain fog, attention disorders
Hormonal: fatigue, sleep problems, depression, anxiety and/or mood swings, menstrual problems, infertility, thyroid problems, osteoporosis/osteopenia
Immune System: frequent infections, arthritis (any type for you or your family), skin problems, autoimmune disease, celiac disease

Non-Celiac gluten sensitivity has been linked to 55 diseases. (*Farrell RJ, Kelly* CP. *Celiac sprue.* N Engl J Med. *2002*;346:180-188) and 30% of people of European decent carry gene for gluten intolerance (*Green PH,* Jabri B. *Coeliac disease. Lancet* 2003; 362: 383-91), although prevalence is also significant in most other races, except Asian.

Gluten sensitivity can result in damaging the sites in the digestive tract where nutrients are assimilated. The damage may be caused by undigested gluten (*meaning gluten damages the absorption sites and the person can have significant nutritional deficiencies despite eating a great diet and taking the best supplements*). The body can produce reactions to gluten, which may or may not affect the digestive system, but can affect every system in the body.

Even a small amount of gluten (a single molecule) can trigger a response although symptoms exist on a continuum from mild to severe in the majority of cases. It is extremely important to understand that if someone does indeed test positive for gluten sensitivity, it is not something that goes away. A strict gluten-free diet (100%) is the only current treatment and if gluten is re-introduced to the diet, a relapse of the symptoms will usually occur and will usually be more severe.

The overall goal in cases of gluten sensitivity is to

1) relieve symptoms by removing all gluten containing foods from the diet
2) educate and inform about gluten-containing foods
3) heal the intestine and reverse the consequences of poor nutrient absorption
4) eat a variety of healthy gluten-free, whole foods

Maintaining a gluten-free diet can be difficult initially, especially when eating out or traveling. Also support from family members or housemates is important because precautionary measures must be taken to prevent cross-contamination of foods. Gluten-free foods must be stored and prepared separately, cooking and serving utensils must be cleaned carefully prior to use, and a separate toaster must be purchased for breads. It is critical to familiarize oneself with gluten-containing and gluten-free foods; especially when eating out or carefully reading food labels when buying groceries.

Gluten-free grains include (include in moderation): Amaranth, Buckwheat, Corn, Millet, Quinoa, Rice (brown, red, wild), Sorghum, Teff, Oats (must be gluten-free oats). BE CAREFUL that you eat these grains in moderation (2 times a day or less). Avoid highly processed gluten-free grains.

Gluten-containing grains (AVOID 100%): Wheat, Barley, Bulgar, Durum, Einkorn, Emmer, Farina, Kamut, Kasha, Rye, Semolina, Spelt, Triticum

Gluten-Containing Products (AVOID)

- Flour Products: *any products that contain flour, bran, wheat germ, wheat starch or gluten*
  Bleached Flour, Bread Flour, Brown Flour, Cereal Binding, Flour *(normally this is wheat)* Graham Flour, Granary Flour, Strong Flour, Unbleached Flour, Whole-Meal Flour, Wheat Amino Acids, Wheat Bran, Wheat Flour Lipids, Wheat Germ Extract/Glycerides/Oil, Wheat Nuts, Wheat Protein

- Baked Goods: Breads (barley, kamut, oat, rye, pumpernickel, spelt, wheat) Bagels, Biscuits, Breakfast Cereals, Buns, Corn Bread, Crackers, Croutons, Matzos, Muffins, Noodles, Pancakes, Pasta (macaroni, spaghetti, lasagna, etc.), Pizza Crust, Pretzels, Rolls, Waffles

- Breads: Some are advertising themselves as gluten-free which contain oats, spelt, kamut, rye; Look for specifically stated gluten-free breads and then ask your health food store to carry a particular one) or other regional brands.

- Alcohol: Beer, Gin, Tequila (Don Julio), Whiskey, Wine coolers *(some made w/ barley malt)*, Vodkas *(unless made with potatoes)*, Wine (sometimes)

- Chocolate Gluten often added as a thickener and not always listed so look for gluten-free listed on the label

- Condiments: Grain vinegar in ketchup, mayonnaise & mustard is often from wheat

- Breaded Foods: Bread crumbs, meats, dumplings, stuffing, deep-fried (chicken, fish, vegetables, cheese sticks)

- Beverages: Cocoa drinks, Postum, Ovaltine, Coffee substitutes, Instant coffee (*wheat flour sometimes added*)

- Dishes: Couscous, Soba Noodles (*wheat sometimes added*), Tabbouleh/Tabouli, Udon (*wheat noodles*)

- Malt: barley malt, malt extract, malt flavoring, malt syrup, malt vinegar

- Oats* *do not inherently contain gluten but most are processed in plants also using gluten grains that cross-contaminate with gluten so choose gluten-free oats:* www.glutenfreeoats.com; *some amaranth and millet flake cereals contain oats*

- Packaged Mixes: Bouillon Cubes, Gravy, Gravy Cubes

- Processed Wheat (hidden gluten): Dextrimaltose, Disodium Wheatgermamido Peg-2 Sulfosuccinate, Hydrolyzed Wheat Gluten, Hydrolyzed Wheat Protein, Hydrolyzed Wheat Protein Pg-Propyl Silanetriol, Hydrolyzed Wheat Starch, Hydroxypropyltrimonium Hydrolyzed Wheat Protein, Stearyldimoniumhydroxypropyl Hydrolyzed Wheat Protein, Wheat Germamidopropyldimonium Hydroxypropyl Hydrolyzed Wheat Protein

- Salad dressing; *(read the label)*

- Soy: Miso *(some made from barley),* Namu Shoyu, Tamari, Teriyaki Sauce (*unless specified wheat-free on the label*), Soy Sauce

- Seitan (*vegetarian, mock-meats*), Fu *(dried wheat gluten)*

- Soups & Sauces *(flour often added as a thickener and not always listed: look for gluten-free listed on the label or ask the restaurant employees)*

- Sweets: Candy, Cakes, Cookies, Doughnuts, Ice Creams & Cones, Ice Cream sandwiches, Pastries, Pie, Pie Crust, Pop Tarts, Pudding

- Starch: *(starch is added to many processed foods)* Corn Starch, Edible Starch, Food Starch, Modified Food Starch, Modified Starch, Vegetable Starch, Textured Vegetable Protein-TVP *(added to many low-quality canned tunas)*

- Vinegar *(many are grain alcohol derived unless specified gluten-free or from apple cider, balsamic, corn, red wine, rice, ume plum)*

Food Additives:

- Glucose syrup - can be derived from either wheat or corn
- Rice Syrup - may contain barley malt
- Dextrin - could be wheat, unless listed as 'corn dextrin' or maltodextrin which, ironically, is corn
- Malt - derived from barley
- Flavor enhancers - could be malt
- Flavorings & Extracts - most use grain alcohol.
- Caramel Color - could be malt
- Modified Food Starch - could be wheat
- Starch that isn't identified - In the U.S. this is usually corn, but elsewhere could be wheat
- Binders, fillers, excipients, extenders - if not specified
- Fu is dried wheat gluten
- MSG is monosodium glutamate. Note that yeast extracts (e.g. Marmite) contain MSG
- HVP (Hydrolized Vegetable Protein) - could be wheat based, ask manufacturer
- HPP is hydrolized plant protein

- TPP is textured plant protein
- TVP is textured vegetable. protein
- Gums such as xantham, guar and pectin, which are used to replace gluten in GF baking, are safe from a gluten viewpoint, but many people with damaged guts find them difficult to digest.

GLUTEN CONTAINING ALCOHOL *(beware of beer and grain alcohol)*

Beer, Gin, Tequila (Don Julio), Whiskey, Wine-coolers *(some made w/ barley malt)*, Vodkas *(unless made with potatoes)*

GLUTEN FREE ALCOHOL:

Beer: Bard's Tale Beer www.bardsbeer.com Dragon's Gold, La Messagere, Green's Explorer, Lakefront New Grist www.lakefrontbrewery.com RedBridge www.redbridgebeer.com Ramapo Valley Brewery:Passover Honey www.ramapovalleybrewery.com, Woodchuck Draft Cider www.woodchuck.com

Liquor: Mead, Rum. Sake *(most)*,Tequila

Wine or Grape-based: Armagnac, Brandy, Champagne, Grappa, Ouzo, Port, Sherry, Sparkling Wine *(note some wine may contain gluten if wine barrels seams use a gluten-based glue which can leach into the wine)*

Other Gluten-free:

- Cider *(most fermented from fruit but some add barley - read labels)* Kirschwasser *(cherry liqueur)*
- Gin *(made from Juniper berries ONLY; most have other grain alcohol added)*
- Martini:
  - *Club Extra Dry Martini (corn & grape)*
  - *Club Vodka Martini (corn & grape)*
- Mead *(distilled from honey)*
- Mixes:
  - *Club Tom Collins* (corn).

- - *Dimond Jims Bloody Mary Mystery.*
  - *Holland House* - all EXCEPT Teriyaki Marinade and Smooth & Spicy Bloody Mary Mixes.
  - *Margarita Jose Cuervo. Mr. & Mrs. T.*
  - *Mr. & Mrs. T* - all Except Bloody Mary Mix.
  - *Spice Islands* - Cooking Wines - Burgundy, Sherry and White.
- Rum
- Sake *(fermented with rice and Koji enzymes. The Koji enzymes are grown on Miso, which is usually made with barley. The two-product separation from barley, and the manufacturing process should make it safe)*
- Tequila: any 100% Agave, Cazadores *Reposado*, Jose Cuervo, Sauza, Cabo Wabo, White Tequila (Albertson's, Acme, Jewel, Equaline Good Day Labels) (Don Julio *NOT gluten-free*)
- Vermouth *(distilled from grapes)*
- Wine: Armagnac, Brandy, Champagne, Grappa, Port, Sherry, Sparkling Wine, Ouzo (*grapes and anise*)
- Vodkas:, Adamba, Blue Ice, Bushman's, Chopin, Cold River Vodka, Ciroc, Hampton's, Jankill, Jinro Soju, Kamachatka, Luksusowa, Monopolowa, Nisskosher Polish, Peconika, Popov Citrus & Popov Tangerine, Reisk, Tito's, Smirnoff Red Label, Smirnoff Citrus Twist, Teton Glacier, Victory, Zodiac
- Wine Coolers:
  - *Bartle & James* wine-based beverages (*not malt beverages - read labels*)
  - *Boones* wine-based beverages (*not malt beverages - read labels*)

Gluten Resources:

www.glutenfreesociety.com

www.celiac.com

www.glutefreewatchdog.com

www.glutenfreemall.com

Drug Mugger List

Cholesterol-Lowering Drugs	
Baycol, Lescol, Lipitor, Mevacor, Zocor	Co Q10, selenium, zinc copper
Colestid, Questran	Magnesium, phosphorus, zinc, vitamins A, B12, E, D, K, folic acid, iron, calcium
Lopid, Tricor	Coenzyme Q10, Vit E
Diuretics	
Loop, Thiazide, Potassium Sparing, Misc.	Vitamin B1, vitamin B6, magnesium, potassium, zinc, vitamin C, folic acid, calcium
Female Hormones	
Estrogen/HRT: Evista, Prempro, Premarin, Estratab	Vitamin B6, vitamin B12, Co Q10, zinc, folic acid, vitamin C, magnesium
Oral Contraceptives: Estrastep, Norinyl, Ortho-Novem, Triphasil	Vitamin B2, vitamin B6, vitamin B12, folic acid, vitamin C, magnesium, zinc
Laxatives	Potassium
Tranquilizers	
Major: Haldol, Vesprin	Vitamin B2, coenzyme Q10
Minor: Lunesta, Ambien	
Psychotherapeutics: Ormazine, Thorazine	
Anti-Convulsants	
Barbituates: Butalan, Brevital, Pentothal	Folic acid, vitamin D, vitamin K, calcium
Phenytoin: Dilantin	Biotin, folic acid, vitamin D, Calcium, vitamin B1, vitamin B12
Carbamazepine: Tegretol	Biotin, folic acid, vitamin D
Bronchodilators	
Theophylline	Vitamin B6
Synthetic Thyroid	Calcium

Drug Induced Nutrient Depletion Handbook, by R. Pelton et al; Physicians Desk Reference

ABOUT THE AUTHOR

Donna Parker LAc. is a Classical Five Element acupuncturist, Certified in Integrative Nutrition, and a Certified Health Coach. She helps busy people create a healthy lifestyle using simple techniques that result in increased vitality and health. She lives in West Marin with her husband, son, and several animals.

www.ingramcontent.com/pod-product-compliance
Lightning Source LLC
Chambersburg PA
CBHW050400290526
45786CB00003B/1060